MASTERING PLUGGED DUCTS IN BREASTFEEDING

A COMPLETE MANUAL FOR PREVENTION AND REMEDY

Alice Brendan

INTRODUCTION 7

CHAPTER 1: UNDERSTANDING PLUGGED MILK DUCTS: 9

The Anatomy of a Plugged Milk Duct: What You Need to Know 13

Recognizing the Signs and Symptoms 19

CHAPTER 2: COMMON CAUSES OF PLUGGED MILK DUCTS AND HOW TO AVOID THEM 22

Preventative Measures: Tips for Keeping Milk Ducts Clear Preventative 27

The Importance of Proper Breastfeeding Techniques in Preventing Plugged Ducts 30

CHAPTER3: WHEN TO SEEK HELP: KNOWING WHEN A PLUGGED DUCT REQUIRES MEDICAL ATTENTION 34

Treatment Options for Plugged Milk Ducts: From Home Remedies to Medical Interventions 38

The Role of Massage and Heat Therapy in Clearing Plugged Milk Ducts 42

CHAPTER4: DIETARY CHANGES AND SUPPLEMENTS FOR PREVENTING PLUGGED DUCTS 46

The Emotional Impact of Plugged Milk Ducts..49

Balancing Work and Breastfeeding...52

CHAPTER5: THE CONNECTION BETWEEN MASTITIS AND PLUGGED MILK DUCTS..55

Navigating the Challenges of Breastfeeding with Plugged Ducts............58

How to Clear Plugged Milk Ducts Quickly and Effectively....................63

CHAPTER6: THE BENEFITS OF LECITHIN SUPPLEMENTS IN PREVENTING PLUGGED DUCTS67

Understanding the Role of Hormones in Plugged Milk Ducts.................71

The Link Between Engorgement and Plugged Ducts: How to Find Relief
....73

CHAPTER7: LIFESTYLE CHANGES FOR........................77

PREVENTING PLUGGED MILK DUCTS IN THE LONG TERM...77

The Impact of Stress on Milk Production and Duct Health The Impact of Stress on Milk Production and Duct Health..82

THE CONNECTION BETWEEN BREASTFEEDING POSITIONS AND PLUGGED DUCTS..85

CHAPTER8: THE ROLE OF LATCHING........................88

TECHNIQUES IN PREVENTING PLUGGED MILK DUCTS **88**

The Benefits of Breastfeeding on Demand **92**

The Importance of Proper Breast Pumping Techniques in Preventing Plugged Ducts **95**

CHAPTER 9: HOW TO MANAGE PLUGGED MILK DUCTS WHILE TRAVELING **99**

The Benefits of Regular Breast Exams in Preventing Plugged Ducts ... **103**

The Connection Between Breastfeeding Frequency and Plugged Ducts **106**

CHAPTER 10: THE IMPACT OF MEDICATIONS ON MILK PRODUCTION AND DUCT HEALTH **109**

The Link Between Allergies and Plugged Milk Ducts **113**

The Role of Blocked Nipples in Plugged Ducts **116**

CHAPTER11: THE BENEFITS OF WARM COMPRESSES IN CLEARING PLUGGED MILK DUCTS **119**

The Connection Between Clogged Milk Ducts and Breast Infections ... **122**

The Impact of Inadequate Milk Supply on Plugged Ducts **126**

CHAPTER 12: THE BENEFITS OF PROPER HYDRATION IN PREVENTING PLUGGED DUCTS .. **128**

The Role of Breastfeeding Support Groups in Preventing Plugged Ducts

.... 131

The Connection Between Breast Engorgement and Plugged Ducts 135

CHAPTER13: THE IMPACT OF ILLNESS ON MILK PRODUCTION AND DUCT HEALTH 137

The Benefits of Massage Oils in Clearing Plugged Milk Ducts 140

The Role of Herbal Remedies in Preventing Plugged Ducts 143

CHAPTER14: THE CONNECTION BETWEEN PLUGGED MILK DUCTS AND BREASTFEEDING SUCCESS 147

CONCLUSION.. 151

BIOGRAPHY 153

Introduction

Welcome to "**Mastering Plugged Ducts in Breastfeeding: A Complete Manual for Prevention and Remedy**" - your ultimate resource for navigating the twists and turns of the breastfeeding journey with confidence and ease.

As mothers, we embark on a sacred journey filled with love, nurturing, and boundless dedication to our little ones' well-being. Yet, amidst the joy of nurturing our babies, we may encounter roadblocks along the way. Plugged milk ducts, a common challenge faced by breastfeeding mothers, can cast a shadow on this beautiful journey, causing discomfort and frustration.

But fear not, dear reader, for within the pages of this ebook lies a treasure trove of wisdom, insights, and practical strategies to help you overcome these obstacles and reclaim the joy of breastfeeding. From understanding the causes of plugged ducts to discovering effective prevention methods and powerful remedies for clearing them, "Unblocking the Path" is your trusted companion on the path to seamless lactation.

Through expert guidance and nurturing remedies, you'll embark on a journey of empowerment, equipped with the knowledge and tools to navigate through any challenges that may arise. Whether you're a first-time mother embarking on the adventure of breastfeeding or a seasoned parent seeking solutions to recurring issues, this ebook is tailored to meet your needs and support you every step of the way.

Join us as we delve into the intricacies of breastfeeding, explore the wonders of maternal wellness, and celebrate the profound bond between mother and child. Let "Unblocking the Path" be your guiding light on this transformative journey, igniting a sense of confidence, empowerment, and joy as you nurture your precious little one.

Dive into the chapters that follow, and unlock the secrets to a fulfilling and rewarding breastfeeding experience. Together, let us embark on this journey with courage, determination, and an unwavering commitment to the health and happiness of both mother and baby.

Chapter 1: Understanding Plugged Milk Ducts:

Breastfeeding embodies a natural bond between mother and baby, offering a plethora of benefits. Yet, amidst its beauty lies the challenge of plugged milk ducts, a common hurdle for nursing mothers. These obstructions can cause discomfort and pain, disrupting the nurturing experience.

Understanding Plugged Milk Ducts:

Plugged milk ducts emerge when the natural flow of milk within a duct is hindered, resulting in accumulation and subsequent inflammation. Particularly prevalent during the initial stages of breastfeeding, when supply and demand are in flux, they manifest as painful swellings.

Indicators of Plugged Milk Ducts:

Detecting plugged milk ducts hinges on recognizing various symptoms, which may differ among individuals:

- Presence of a painful lump or hardened area in the breast.
- Notable redness and swelling in the affected region.
- Sensation of fullness or engorgement in the breast.
- Experience of pain or tenderness, particularly during breastfeeding or pumping sessions.
- Decline in milk supply from the affected breast.

Root Causes of Plugged Milk Ducts:

Several factors contribute to the onset of plugged milk ducts, including:

- Inadequate or irregular emptying of the breast: Failure to fully empty the breast during nursing or pumping can cause milk accumulation and subsequent blockage in the ducts.

- External pressure on the breast: Tight-fitting clothing or bras, sleeping positions that compress the breasts, or carrying heavy loads on one shoulder can exert pressure on the ducts, leading to blockages.

- Suboptimal latch or positioning: Incorrect latch by the baby or improper breastfeeding posture can impede effective milk expulsion, paving the way for plugged ducts.

- Stress or fatigue: Psychological stress or exhaustion can disrupt milk production and flow, heightening the risk of plugged ducts.

- Potential progression to mastitis: In some cases, plugged ducts may evolve into mastitis, a more severe condition characterized by breast tissue infection.

Preventing and Treating Plugged Milk Ducts:

Navigating the journey of breastfeeding can encounter the hurdle of plugged milk ducts, but proactive measures can mitigate their occurrence. Here's how to prevent and manage them effectively:

Preventive Measures:

- Maintain frequent breastfeeding sessions: Encouraging regular and efficient feeding sessions aids in preventing milk accumulation within the ducts.

- Ensure correct latch: Prioritize correct latching techniques and optimal breastfeeding positions to facilitate effective milk drainage.

- Opt for loose attire: Embrace loose and comfortable clothing choices to alleviate pressure on the ducts.

- Self-care regimen: Prioritize adequate rest, hydration, and stress management to foster optimal milk production and flow.

Treatment Strategies:

- Continue breastfeeding or pumping: Sustaining breastfeeding or pumping from the affected breast helps in alleviating the blockage and associated discomfort. Ensure thorough and frequent emptying of the breast.

- Apply warm compress: Prior to feeding or pumping, applying a warm compress to the affected breast aids in loosening the blockage and promoting milk flow.

- Gentle massage: Incorporate gentle massage techniques during breastfeeding or pumping sessions to disperse the blockage and stimulate milk flow.

- Prioritize rest and hydration: Optimal rest and hydration levels support healthy milk production and flow, aiding in resolving the issue.

- Over-the-counter pain relief: In cases of discomfort, consider over-the-counter pain relievers such as ibuprofen to alleviate pain and inflammation.

Knowing When to Seek Assistance:

While home management is effective for most instances of plugged milk ducts, certain signs warrant medical attention:

- Persistent symptoms despite home treatments.
- Development of fever or flu-like symptoms.
- Presence of unusual discharge or changes in breast appearance.
- Concerns regarding the baby's feeding patterns or well-being.

Seeking timely medical assistance ensures comprehensive management and resolution of plugged milk ducts, fostering a smoother breastfeeding journey.

Recognizing Signs of Concern:

- Lack of improvement with home remedies.

- Onset of fever or flu-like symptoms.
- Escalation in redness, heat, or swelling of the affected breast.
- Observation of pus or blood in breast milk.

Prompt Action is Key:

If any of these symptoms manifest, reaching out to your healthcare provider promptly is essential for thorough assessment and appropriate intervention.

In Summary:

Plugged milk ducts, while common, are typically manageable for breastfeeding mothers. Equipping yourself with knowledge about their causes, symptoms, and treatments empowers you to navigate this challenge adeptly, ensuring uninterrupted enjoyment of the myriad benefits breastfeeding offers for both you and your baby.

The Anatomy of a Plugged Milk Duct: What You Need to Know

Exploring Plugged Milk Ducts: Understanding, Causes, and Management

Plugged milk ducts, also referred to as blocked or clogged milk ducts, are a common concern encountered during breastfeeding. They occur when milk isn't adequately drained from the breast, resulting in the accumulation of milk, leading to discomfort and inflammation.

In this discussion, we delve into the intricacies of plugged milk ducts, including their anatomy, causes, and effective management strategies.

Anatomy of Plugged Milk Ducts:

Understanding the anatomy of a plugged milk duct begins with comprehending how milk production and storage occur within the breast. The breast comprises glandular tissue housing milk-producing cells called alveoli.

 These alveoli are connected to small ducts responsible for transporting milk to the nipple for breastfeeding.

During feeding sessions, milk is released from the alveoli into the ducts, ultimately exiting through the nipple. However, when milk isn't efficiently drained, it can lead to the formation of a plugged milk duct. Several factors contribute to this, including:

- Infrequent or incomplete feedings: Irregular or insufficient feedings can result in milk accumulation within the ducts, causing blockages.

- Pressure on the breast: External factors such as tight clothing, ill-fitting bras, or sleeping positions can exert pressure on breast tissue, hindering milk flow and causing blockages.

- Engorgement: Overfilling of the breasts with milk can exert pressure on the ducts, leading to blockages.

- Poor latch: Inadequate latching during breastfeeding prevents effective milk flow, contributing to plugged ducts.

- Stress or fatigue: Psychological stress and fatigue can disrupt milk production and letdown, increasing the likelihood of plugged ducts.

Symptoms of Plugged Milk Ducts:

Symptoms of plugged milk ducts can manifest differently in individuals, but common indicators include:

- Pain, tenderness, or swelling in the breast.
- Presence of a lump or hard knot in the breast.
- Redness or warmth in the affected area.
- Decreased milk supply from the affected breast.
- Sensation of burning or stinging during breastfeeding.
- Onset of fever or flu-like symptoms.

Seeking Assistance:

If experiencing any of these symptoms, seeking guidance from a healthcare provider or lactation consultant is crucial for accurate diagnosis and appropriate treatment.

Plugged milk ducts pose a common challenge for breastfeeding mothers, but understanding their anatomy, causes, and symptoms enables effective management and prevention. By promptly addressing concerns and seeking professional support when needed, mothers can navigate this aspect of breastfeeding with confidence and ensure continued nurturing for both themselves and their baby.

Addressing Plugged Milk Ducts: Effective Treatments and Prevention Strategies

Plugged milk ducts pose discomfort for breastfeeding mothers but can be effectively managed with various treatments. Additionally, implementing preventive measures can reduce the likelihood of occurrence. This discussion explores treatment options and preventive strategies for plugged milk ducts.

Treatment Options:

Several methods can alleviate symptoms and clear plugged milk ducts:

- Breastfeeding: Continued breastfeeding from the affected breast aids in clearing the blockage. Positioning your baby to ensure their chin points towards the blocked duct facilitates efficient milk drainage.

- Massage: Gentle massage of the affected area during breastfeeding or pumping helps disperse the blockage and stimulate milk flow.

- Warm compress: Application of a warm compress to the affected breast before breastfeeding or pumping softens the blockage, easing its clearance.

- Cold compress: Post-feeding or pumping, applying a cold compress reduces inflammation and alleviates pain.

- Rest and hydration: Adequate rest and hydration support the body's ability to clear the blockage and reduce inflammation.

Seeking Further Intervention:

If the plugged milk duct persists despite home remedies or if concerning symptoms such as fever develop, seeking medical assistance is crucial. Additional treatments may include:

- Antibiotics: In cases of infection, antibiotics are prescribed to clear the infection.

- Ultrasound therapy: Utilized to break up the blockage and promote milk flow.

- Surgical intervention: Rarely, surgical removal of the blockage may be necessary.

Prevention Strategies:

Implementing preventive measures reduces the risk of plugged milk ducts:

- Breastfeed frequently: On-demand feeding ensures effective breast drainage, preventing milk buildup in the ducts.
- Ensure proper latch: Proper latch promotes efficient milk flow, reducing the likelihood of blockages.
- Avoid tight clothing: Opt for loose, comfortable attire and a well-fitting bra to alleviate pressure on breast tissue.
- Prioritize rest and relaxation: Adequate rest and stress management contribute to overall breast health.

By employing effective treatments and preventive strategies, breastfeeding mothers can navigate plugged milk ducts with confidence, ensuring a smooth breastfeeding journey for both mother and baby.

Recognizing the Signs and Symptoms

Breastfeeding is a wonderful and natural way to nourish your baby, but it can come with its own set of challenges. One common issue that many breastfeeding moms face is plugged milk ducts.

Plugged milk ducts occur when milk is not effectively removed from the breast, leading to a blockage in the milk duct. This can be painful and uncomfortable, but with proper recognition and treatment, plugged milk ducts can be resolved quickly.

In this article, we will discuss the signs and symptoms of plugged milk ducts, as well as some tips on how to prevent and treat them.

Signs and Symptoms of Plugged Milk Ducts

1.   Pain and tenderness: One of the most common signs of a plugged milk duct is pain and tenderness in the affected breast. This pain is often localized to a specific area of the breast and may feel like a sharp or throbbing sensation. The breast may also feel tender to the touch.

2.   Swelling and redness: Plugged milk ducts can cause the affected breast to become swollen and red. This swelling and redness may be accompanied by a feeling of warmth in the breast.

3.   Lumps or hard spots: Plugged milk ducts can cause lumps or hard spots to form in the breast. These lumps may be

painful to the touch and can vary in size.

4.   Decreased milk flow: Another sign of a plugged milk duct is a decrease in milk flow from the affected breast. This can result in your baby having difficulty latching or not getting enough milk during feedings.

5.   Engorgement: Plugged milk ducts can also lead to engorgement in the affected breast. Engorgement occurs when the breast becomes overfilled with milk, causing it to feel heavy and uncomfortable.

6.   Fever and flu-like symptoms: In some cases, plugged milk ducts can cause a low-grade fever and flu-like symptoms, such as fatigue and body aches. If you experience these symptoms along with the other signs of a plugged milk duct, it is important to seek medical attention.

Preventing Plugged Milk Ducts

While plugged milk ducts can be a common occurrence for breastfeeding moms, there are some steps you can take to help prevent them from happening:

1.   Ensure proper latch: A proper latch is essential for effective milk removal and can help prevent plugged milk ducts. Make sure your baby is latching correctly and seek help from a lactation consultant if needed.

2.   Empty the breast completely: Make sure to empty your

breasts completely during feedings to prevent milk from backing up in the ducts. If your baby is not emptying the breast, consider pumping after feedings to ensure thorough emptying.

3.   Avoid tight clothing: Tight clothing, such as bras or shirts, can restrict milk flow and contribute to plugged milk ducts. Opt for loose-fitting clothing that allows for proper milk flow.

4.   Stay hydrated: Drinking plenty of water can help keep your milk flowing smoothly and prevent blockages in the ducts. Aim to drink at least eight glasses of water a day.

5.   Massage the breasts: Massaging your breasts before and during feedings can help stimulate milk flow and prevent plugged milk ducts. Gently massage the affected breast in a circular motion to help release any blockages.

Treating Plugged Milk Ducts

If you suspect you have a plugged milk duct, there are several things you can do to help relieve the symptoms and clear the blockage:

1.   Nurse frequently: The best way to clear a plugged milk duct is to nurse frequently from the affected breast. Make sure your baby is latching correctly and try different nursing positions to help drain the breast thoroughly.

2.   Apply heat: Applying heat to the affected breast can help loosen the blockage and relieve pain and swelling. You can use a warm compress, a heating pad, or take a warm shower to help

alleviate symptoms.

3.   Massage the breast: Gently massaging the affected breast can help break up the blockage and promote milk flow. Use gentle circular motions to massage the breast and focus on the area where the blockage is located.

4.   Pump or hand express: If your baby is having difficulty latching or draining the breast, consider pumping or hand expressing milk to help clear the blockage. Pumping can help remove milk more efficiently and prevent further blockages.

5.   Rest and relax: Stress and fatigue can contribute to plugged milk ducts, so it is important to rest and relax as much as possible. Take breaks throughout the day, practice deep breathing exercises, and ask for help from friends and family members.

When to Seek Medical Attention

In most cases, plugged milk ducts can be resolved at home with the above treatments. However, there are some situations where you should seek medical attention:

- If you have a fever higher than 101 degrees

Chapter 2: Common Causes of Plugged Milk Ducts and How to Avoid Them

While breastfeeding is a cherished experience, it's not without its hurdles. Plugged milk ducts are a common challenge faced by many mothers. These blockages can cause discomfort and, if left untreated, may escalate to more serious issues like mastitis.

This article aims to shed light on the common causes of plugged milk ducts and offer practical tips to prevent them.

Common Causes of Plugged Milk Ducts:

1. Poor Latch: A leading cause of plugged milk ducts is a poor latch. When a baby doesn't latch correctly onto the breast, milk flow is hindered, leading to milk backup in the ducts and eventual blockage. Seeking guidance from a lactation consultant can help ensure proper latching technique.

2. Infrequent Feedings: Infrequent feedings contribute to plugged milk ducts by allowing milk to accumulate in the ducts. Feeding your baby on demand and as frequently as needed helps maintain milk flow and prevents blockages from forming.

3. Tight Clothing: Wearing tight clothing, particularly bras, can exert pressure on the breasts, impeding milk flow and causing blockages. Opting for comfortable, supportive bras that don't constrict breast tissue can mitigate this risk.

4. Poor Breastfeeding Position: The breastfeeding position plays a pivotal role in preventing plugged milk ducts. Consistently breastfeeding in a position that applies undue pressure to specific areas of the breast can lead to

blockages. Experimenting with different positions and using supportive aids can alleviate this issue.

Prevention Strategies:

By implementing preventive measures, you can reduce the likelihood of encountering plugged milk ducts:

- Prioritize proper latch techniques.
- Feed your baby on demand to maintain milk flow.
- Opt for comfortable, supportive clothing.
- Explore various breastfeeding positions for optimal comfort.

Understanding the causes of plugged milk ducts and adopting preventive strategies empowers breastfeeding mothers to navigate this aspect of breastfeeding with ease. By addressing potential risk factors and embracing techniques to promote optimal milk flow, mothers can enjoy a fulfilling breastfeeding journey with their babies.

Exploring Factors Contributing to Plugged Milk Ducts

Plugged milk ducts present a common challenge for breastfeeding mothers, influenced by various factors. Understanding these contributors is crucial for effective prevention. This discussion delves into the key factors that can lead to plugged milk ducts and offers insights into mitigating their impact.

1. Stress:

Stress exerts a significant influence on breastfeeding, potentially contributing to plugged milk ducts. Elevated stress levels trigger hormone release, affecting milk production and flow, thus increasing the risk of duct blockages. To mitigate this, prioritize stress reduction through relaxation techniques, ample rest, and seeking support from loved ones.

2. Dehydration:

Inadequate hydration is another factor implicated in plugged milk ducts. Insufficient fluid intake results in denser, more concentrated milk, predisposing to duct blockages. Maintaining adequate hydration by drinking plenty of water throughout the day is essential. Additionally, herbal teas or hydrating beverages can supplement fluid intake effectively.

3. Poor Breast Emptying:

Incomplete breast emptying during feedings can lead to milk backup in the ducts, fostering plugged ducts. This may occur due to ineffective feeding or inadequate pumping. Ensuring thorough breast emptying by allowing your baby to nurse on both sides and employing breast compression techniques promotes optimal milk flow, reducing the risk of blockages.

4. Early Introduction of Pacifiers or Bottles:

Introducing pacifiers or bottles prematurely may hinder effective breastfeeding, potentially leading to plugged milk ducts. When babies use pacifiers or bottles, they may not nurse as efficiently at the breast, resulting in milk accumulation in the ducts.

Delaying the introduction of pacifiers or bottles until breastfeeding is well-established minimizes this risk. If needed, use them sparingly while prioritizing breastfeeding.

5. Engorgement:

Breast engorgement, characterized by excessive milk accumulation, poses a risk for plugged milk ducts. Engorged breasts impede milk flow, predisposing to duct blockages. Preventing engorgement through frequent nursing and cold compresses or cabbage leaves to alleviate swelling mitigates this risk effectively.

6. Ill-Fitting Breast Pump:

Using an ill-fitting or malfunctioning breast pump can also contribute to plugged milk ducts. Improperly fitting pumps may cause uneven suction, leading to duct blockages. Opting for a properly fitting breast pump and ensuring its functionality is essential for preventing this issue.

Awareness of these factors influencing plugged milk ducts empowers breastfeeding mothers to take proactive measures for prevention. By addressing these contributors and adopting preventive strategies, mothers can enhance their breastfeeding experience and minimize the risk of encountering plugged milk ducts.

**Preventative Measures: Tips for Keeping Milk Ducts Clear
Preventative**

Breastfeeding is a cherished journey, yet it presents challenges, with blocked milk ducts being a prevalent issue. Addressing this concern promptly is vital to ensure a smooth breastfeeding experience. This article delves into preventive measures and tips to maintain clear milk ducts, enhancing your breastfeeding journey.

Understanding Milk Ducts:

Milk ducts are intricate channels that transport milk from breast cells to the nipple. Blockages in these ducts can lead to discomfort and swelling, potentially progressing to mastitis—an infection of the breast tissue. Prioritizing preventive measures is crucial to prevent such complications.

Preventive Measures for Clearing Milk Ducts:

1. Master Proper Latching Technique:

Ensuring a correct latch during breastfeeding is paramount to prevent blocked milk ducts. A poor latch impedes milk removal efficiency, increasing the risk of blockages. Seek assistance from a lactation consultant if you experience breastfeeding discomfort, as improving latch technique is key to preventing blocked ducts.

2. Embrace Frequent Breastfeeding:

Regular breastfeeding sessions facilitate continuous milk flow, preventing milk stagnation in the ducts—a precursor to blockages. Feed your baby on demand to ensure frequent breast emptying, reducing the likelihood of blocked ducts. Consider pumping if necessary to maintain milk flow and prevent blockages.

3. Ensure Complete Breast Emptying:

Thorough breast emptying during each feeding session is imperative to prevent blocked ducts. Utilize a breast pump to express any residual milk if your baby doesn't fully drain the breast. Leaving milk in the breast heightens the risk of blockages, emphasizing the importance of regular breast emptying.

Proactively implementing preventive measures is essential for maintaining clear milk ducts and fostering a smooth breastfeeding journey. By prioritizing proper latch technique, embracing frequent breastfeeding, and ensuring complete breast emptying, breastfeeding mothers can mitigate the risk of encountering blocked milk ducts. Embrace these tips to enhance your breastfeeding experience and nurture a strong bond with your baby.

Strategies for Preventing Blocked Milk Ducts

1. Opt for Comfort:

Avoid tight clothing and underwire bras that can compress the milk ducts, impeding milk flow and leading to blockages. Choose loose-fitting, comfortable attire and bras without underwire to facilitate proper milk flow. Steer clear of tight straps or bands that may constrict the breasts and increase the risk of blockages.

2. Embrace Massage and Warm Compress:

Incorporate breast massage into your routine before and during breastfeeding to alleviate blockages and enhance milk flow. Utilize gentle circular motions, directing towards the nipple, to encourage unhindered milk flow. Additionally, apply a warm compress to the affected breast to alleviate pain and inflammation associated with blocked ducts.

3. Prioritize Hydration and Nutrition:

Maintain optimal breast health by staying hydrated and consuming a nutritious diet. Ensure adequate water intake throughout the day to prevent blockages. Opt for a balanced diet comprising fruits, vegetables, whole grains, and lean proteins to support milk production and promote breast health.

4. Manage Stress:

Combat stress, a potential deterrent to milk production, by incorporating relaxation techniques into your daily routine. Practice deep breathing, meditation, or yoga to alleviate stress. Allocate time for self-care to rest and rejuvenate, seeking support from loved ones or healthcare providers if needed.

5. Adopt Proper Breastfeeding Positions:

Enhance milk flow and promote a correct latch by experimenting with various breastfeeding positions. Explore options such as the football hold, cradle hold, or side-lying position to determine what works best for you and your baby. Ensure your baby's head is aligned with their body, and their nose faces the nipple for optimal latch.

6. Address Breastfeeding Challenges Promptly:

Promptly address any breastfeeding difficulties, such as pain or inadequate milk supply, to prevent blocked ducts. Seek assistance from lactation consultants or healthcare providers to resolve issues early on. Early intervention can prevent complications and maintain clear milk ducts.

7. Monitor Breast Health:

Regularly monitor your breasts for signs of blockages, including painful lumps, swelling, or redness. Take immediate action if any symptoms arise, such as applying warm compresses, massaging the affected area, and continuing breastfeeding or pumping to alleviate blockages and ensure clear milk ducts.

The Importance of Proper Breastfeeding Techniques in Preventing Plugged Ducts

Breastfeeding is a natural and beautiful way to nourish your baby, but it can also come with its fair share of challenges. One common issue that many breastfeeding mothers face is plugged ducts.

Plugged ducts occur when milk is not properly drained from the breast, leading to a blockage in the milk duct. This can be painful and uncomfortable for the mother, and if not addressed promptly, can lead to more serious complications such as mastitis.

Proper breastfeeding techniques are essential in preventing plugged ducts and ensuring a smooth and successful breastfeeding experience for both mother and baby. In this article, we will discuss the importance of proper breastfeeding techniques in preventing plugged ducts, as well as some tips and strategies for avoiding this common breastfeeding issue.

One of the most important aspects of proper breastfeeding technique is ensuring that your baby is latched on correctly. A proper latch is crucial for effective milk transfer and drainage, which helps to prevent plugged ducts.

When your baby is latched on correctly, their mouth should be wide open, with their lips flanged outwards and their chin pressed into the breast. Their nose should be touching your breast, and their tongue should be extended over their lower gumline.

If your baby is not latched on correctly, they may not be able to effectively drain the breast, leading to a buildup of milk and a potential plugged duct.

If you are experiencing pain or discomfort while breastfeeding, it is important to seek help from a lactation consultant or other breastfeeding support professional to ensure that your baby is latched on correctly.

Another important aspect of proper breastfeeding technique is ensuring that your baby is feeding frequently and effectively. Frequent feeding helps to ensure that your breasts are regularly emptied of milk, reducing the risk of plugged ducts.

It is important to feed your baby on demand, rather than on a strict schedule, as this can help to prevent engorgement and ensure that your breasts are adequately drained.

In addition to feeding frequently, it is also important to ensure that your baby is effectively draining each breast during each feeding session.

This can be achieved by allowing your baby to feed on one breast until it is fully drained before offering the other breast. If your baby is not draining the breast completely, you can try massaging the breast or using gentle compression to help facilitate milk flow.

Proper positioning is also key in preventing plugged ducts. It is important to find a comfortable and supportive position for breastfeeding that allows your baby to latch on correctly and effectively drain the breast.

Some common breastfeeding positions include the cradle hold, football hold, and side-lying position. Experiment with different positions to find what works best for you and your baby.

In addition to proper breastfeeding techniques, there are some other strategies that can help to prevent plugged ducts. One important tip is to ensure that you are adequately hydrated and well-nourished.

Drinking plenty of water and eating a balanced diet can help to ensure that your body is producing an adequate supply of milk and that your breasts are properly drained.

It is also important to avoid tight-fitting clothing or bras that can restrict milk flow and lead to plugged ducts. Opt for loose, comfortable clothing and bras that provide adequate support without constricting your breasts. You may also find relief from plugged ducts by applying warm compresses to the affected breast or taking a warm shower to help facilitate milk flow.

If you do develop a plugged duct, it is important to address it promptly to prevent more serious complications such as mastitis. Some common strategies for treating plugged ducts include massaging the affected area, applying heat, and breastfeeding or pumping frequently to help clear the blockage.

 If you are unable to clear the plugged duct on your own, it is important to seek help from a healthcare provider or lactation consultant for further guidance.

In conclusion, proper breastfeeding techniques are essential in preventing plugged ducts and ensuring a successful breastfeeding experience for both mother and baby.

By following the tips and strategies outlined in this article, you can help to reduce your risk of developing plugged ducts and enjoy a smooth and comfortable breastfeeding journey.

Remember to seek help from a healthcare provider or lactation consultant if you are experiencing pain or discomfort while breastfeeding, as they can provide valuable support and guidance to help you overcome any challenges you may face.

Chapter3: When to Seek Help: Knowing When a Plugged Duct Requires Medical Attention

While breastfeeding is a natural and enriching experience, it can also present challenges like plugged ducts. Understanding the signs, seeking timely assistance, and adopting preventive measures are crucial for managing this issue effectively.

This article explores the signs and symptoms of plugged ducts, when to seek medical attention, and strategies for prevention.

Identifying Signs and Symptoms:

Plugged ducts manifest in various ways, including:

- Tender or painful lump in the breast
- Redness or warmth in the affected area

- Breast swelling or engorgement
- Sensation of fullness or heaviness in the breast
- Decrease in milk supply from the affected breast
- Flu-like symptoms such as fever or chills

Recognizing these signs is essential for prompt intervention to prevent complications like mastitis.

When to Seek Help:

While home remedies like warm compresses and massage are often effective, certain circumstances necessitate medical attention:

- Symptoms persisting beyond 24-48 hours despite home treatment
- Development of a fever of 101.3°F (38.5°C) or higher
- Severe pain or swelling in the breast
- Presence of pus or blood in breast milk
- History of recurrent plugged ducts or mastitis
- Compromised immune system or underlying health conditions

Seeking prompt medical evaluation is crucial in such cases to prevent escalation and ensure proper treatment.

Preventive Strategies:

Taking proactive steps can reduce the risk of plugged ducts:

- Ensure proper breastfeeding techniques, including proper latch and positioning.

- Feed frequently to maintain milk flow and prevent duct blockages.
- Prioritize breast emptying during feedings to prevent milk backup.
- Avoid tight clothing and underwire bras that may constrict milk ducts.
- Manage stress levels through relaxation techniques and self-care practices.
- Maintain hydration and a balanced diet to support breast health.

By recognizing the signs, seeking timely assistance, and adopting preventive measures, breastfeeding mothers can effectively manage plugged ducts and maintain a smooth breastfeeding journey. Embracing these strategies empowers mothers to navigate potential challenges with confidence, ensuring optimal health for both mother and baby.

Preventing Blocked Milk Ducts: Essential Tips for Breastfeeding Mothers

While blocked milk ducts can pose challenges for breastfeeding mothers, adopting preventive measures can significantly reduce the risk of encountering this issue. This article explores practical tips for preventing blocked ducts, ensuring a smoother breastfeeding journey.

Key Strategies for Prevention:

1. Ensure Proper Latch and Positioning:

Optimal latch and positioning during breastfeeding are crucial for effective milk drainage. Ensure that your baby latches onto the breast correctly and maintains a comfortable position to facilitate efficient milk flow.

2. Avoid Tight-Fitting Bras and Clothing:

Steer clear of tight-fitting bras and clothing that may impede milk flow and contribute to blocked ducts. Opt for comfortable, supportive attire that allows for unrestricted milk flow.

3. Maintain Frequent Nursing or Pumping:

Regular nursing or pumping sessions prevent breast engorgement, reducing the likelihood of blocked ducts. Establish a consistent feeding schedule to maintain milk flow and prevent milk backup.

4. Utilize Warm Compresses and Showers:

Prior to nursing or pumping, apply warm compresses to the breasts or indulge in a warm shower. Heat helps to loosen any potential blockages, facilitating smoother milk flow.

5. Incorporate Breast Massage:

During nursing or pumping sessions, incorporate gentle breast massage to break up any clogs and promote milk flow. Massage in circular motions towards the nipple to encourage drainage.

6. Stay Hydrated and Maintain a Balanced Diet:

Hydration and nutrition play vital roles in supporting milk production and breast health. Stay adequately hydrated and consume a balanced diet rich in nutrients to ensure optimal milk supply.

Conclusion:

By implementing these preventive measures, breastfeeding mothers can minimize the risk of encountering blocked milk ducts and enjoy a more comfortable breastfeeding experience.

However, it's crucial to recognize when to seek medical assistance. Persistent symptoms, severe pain, fever, or other concerning signs warrant prompt evaluation and treatment from a healthcare provider.

Prioritize self-care and seek help when needed to safeguard your health and well-being, ensuring a fulfilling breastfeeding journey for both you and your baby.

Treatment Options for Plugged Milk Ducts: From Home Remedies to Medical Interventions

Plugged milk ducts, a common concern among breastfeeding mothers, occur when milk flow is obstructed, leading to discomfort and potential complications. Prompt intervention is crucial to ensure ongoing breastfeeding success. This article delves into treatment options for plugged milk ducts, encompassing both home remedies and medical interventions.

Treatment Options:

Home Remedies:

1. Warm Compress: Ease blockage and promote milk flow by applying a warm compress to the affected breast. Simply dampen a washcloth with warm water, wring it out, and apply it to the breast for 10-15 minutes. Repeat several times daily to alleviate the blockage effectively.

2. Gentle Massage: Break up the blockage and stimulate milk flow through gentle massage. Employ circular motions around the blocked area, directing towards the nipple. Exercise caution to avoid exacerbating inflammation.

3. Ensure Proper Latch: Prevent plugged milk ducts by ensuring your baby latches onto the breast correctly. Ensure their mouth covers as much of the areola as possible, facilitating unhindered milk flow through the ducts.

4. Frequent Nursing: Reduce the likelihood of plugged milk ducts by nursing your baby frequently. Encourage complete breast emptying at each feeding session, thereby preventing milk stagnation within the ducts.

5. Rest and Hydration: Support your body's healing process and prevent further blockages by prioritizing self-care.

Get ample rest, stay hydrated, and maintain a nutritious diet to aid in natural recovery.

By employing these treatment options, breastfeeding mothers can effectively manage plugged milk ducts and alleviate associated discomfort. However, if symptoms persist or worsen, seeking medical advice is essential.

Prompt intervention ensures timely resolution and facilitates continued breastfeeding success. Remember to prioritize self-care and seek professional guidance when needed, ensuring a fulfilling breastfeeding journey for both mother and baby.

Advanced Treatments for Plugged Milk Ducts

1. Ultrasound Therapy: Ultrasound therapy offers a non-invasive approach to address blocked milk ducts. This treatment employs high-frequency sound waves to target and break up the blockage, promoting improved milk flow. By stimulating blood circulation in the affected area, ultrasound therapy aids in resolving the obstruction effectively.

2. Antibiotics: In cases where a plugged milk duct becomes infected, antibiotics may be prescribed to manage the infection. These medications help combat bacterial growth, clearing the infection and preventing its spread. Your healthcare provider will determine the appropriate antibiotic treatment based on the severity of the infection.

3. Consultation with Lactation Consultant: Seeking guidance from a lactation consultant can prove beneficial in managing plugged milk ducts.

   A lactation consultant offers valuable insights into correct breastfeeding techniques, ensuring proper latch and milk flow. Additionally, they provide support and encouragement throughout the recovery process, empowering mothers to navigate this challenge effectively.

4. Manual Expression: When traditional methods fail to resolve a plugged milk duct, manual expression may be necessary. Using gentle massage techniques or a breast pump, mothers can assist in expressing trapped milk from the affected breast. This aids in clearing the blockage and restoring normal milk flow.

5. Surgical Intervention: In rare instances of persistent blocked milk ducts, surgical intervention may be recommended. A surgical procedure can effectively remove the blockage, allowing for unimpeded milk flow. Your healthcare provider will assess the situation and determine if surgical intervention is necessary for resolution.

While dealing with plugged milk ducts can be challenging, effective treatment options are available to provide relief and support breastfeeding mothers.

By incorporating advanced treatments alongside home remedies and seeking guidance from healthcare professionals, mothers can overcome this condition and continue to provide nourishment to their babies.

Remember to prioritize self-care, seek assistance when needed, and approach treatment with confidence, knowing that plugged milk ducts can be effectively managed with the right interventions.

The Role of Massage and Heat Therapy in Clearing Plugged Milk Ducts

Blocked milk ducts, also referred to as plugged milk ducts, pose a common challenge for breastfeeding mothers. This condition arises when one or more milk ducts in the breast become obstructed, impeding the smooth flow of milk.

Without timely intervention, it can lead to discomfort, swelling, and potential infection. Among the various methods available to alleviate plugged milk ducts, massage therapy and heat therapy stand out as natural and effective remedies.

Massage therapy, rooted in ancient healing practices, proves instrumental in promoting healing and relaxation. In the context of resolving plugged milk ducts, massage serves as a potent technique to dislodge the obstruction and stimulate milk flow.

By applying gentle pressure and circular motions to the affected breast, massage helps to loosen the blockage, fostering milk production while mitigating pain, swelling, and the risk of complications like mastitis.

Numerous massage techniques can be employed to address plugged milk ducts. A common approach involves starting from the outer edge of the breast and gradually moving towards the nipple, employing firm yet gentle pressure.

Additionally, a kneading motion, delicately squeezing and releasing the breast, aids in breaking up the blockage. It's crucial to exercise gentleness and avoid excessive pressure to prevent discomfort and potential harm to the breast tissue.

In tandem with massage therapy, heat therapy emerges as another effective strategy for clearing plugged milk ducts. Heat works by relaxing the muscles and tissues in the breast, facilitating milk flow, and reducing pain and swelling.

Warm compresses, hot water bottles, or warm showers serve as viable options for applying heat therapy to the affected breast.

Warm compresses, a popular choice for heat therapy, involve soaking a clean cloth in warm water, wringing out excess water, and placing it on the affected breast for 10-15 minutes. This process can be repeated several times a day to alleviate discomfort and promote milk flow. However, caution must be exercised to ensure the compress is not excessively hot to prevent skin burns or damage.

Another effective approach involves taking a warm shower, allowing the warm water and steam to envelop the breast, relaxing muscles and tissues. Gentle breast massage during the shower further aids in dislodging the blockage and promoting healing.

This method offers a soothing and efficient means of clearing plugged milk ducts.

In addition to massage and heat therapy, proper positioning and latch during breastfeeding play a pivotal role in preventing blocked ducts. Ensuring the baby is positioned correctly and latched onto the breast optimally promotes effective milk flow. Varying breastfeeding positions can aid in clearing blockages and stimulating milk production.

Furthermore, nursing or pumping frequently proves beneficial in preventing milk backup and subsequent blockages. Regularly emptying the breast helps maintain a steady milk supply and reduces the risk of plugged ducts. Attentiveness to the body's signals and the baby's cues ensures adequate nursing or pumping frequency to stave off blockages.

In conclusion, while plugged milk ducts present a common challenge for breastfeeding mothers, effective remedies exist to alleviate discomfort and restore milk flow.

Through the application of massage and heat therapy, coupled with proper breastfeeding practices and frequent nursing or pumping, mothers can effectively manage plugged ducts, ensuring a smooth breastfeeding journey for both themselves and their babies.

In certain instances, over-the-counter solutions like lecithin supplements or herbal remedies may offer assistance in clearing plugged milk ducts. These supplements work by reducing the viscosity of the milk, facilitating smoother milk flow and averting blockages.

However, it's crucial to consult with a healthcare professional before incorporating any supplements or remedies to ascertain their safety and efficacy for both you and your baby.

Should you encounter persistent pain, swelling, or fever associated with plugged milk ducts, seeking medical attention is imperative. In such cases, a healthcare provider might prescribe antibiotics to address any infection or suggest other interventions to clear the blockage.

Swiftly addressing plugged milk ducts is essential to prevent further complications and ensure continued successful breastfeeding for you and your baby.

In summary, employing massage and heat therapy offers effective and natural means to clear plugged milk ducts and stimulate milk flow. By employing gentle massage techniques and applying heat therapy to the affected breast, you can alleviate pain, swelling, and discomfort linked with plugged ducts.

Attentiveness to your body's signals and your baby's cues is key to nursing or pumping frequently enough to stave off blockages.

Should persistent pain or swelling arise, prompt medical attention is advisable. With appropriate care and treatment, resolving plugged milk ducts is achievable.

Chapter4: Dietary Changes and Supplements for Preventing Plugged Ducts

Breastfeeding offers a beautiful connection between mother and baby, yet it's not without its challenges, including the discomfort of plugged ducts.

When a milk duct becomes obstructed, it can result in a painful lump in the breast, causing frustration for nursing mothers. However, dietary adjustments and supplements can play a significant role in preventing this issue.

Staying adequately hydrated is paramount in preventing plugged ducts. Maintaining a steady intake of water throughout the day ensures optimal milk flow and minimizes the risk of blockages. Aim for 8-10 glasses daily, increasing intake while breastfeeding.

Keeping a water bottle nearby serves as a helpful reminder to stay hydrated.

Furthermore, maintaining a balanced diet rich in fruits, vegetables, whole grains, and lean proteins is crucial. Foods abundant in vitamin C, such as oranges and bell peppers, bolster the immune system, warding off infections that could lead to plugged ducts. Similarly, omega-3 fatty acids found in salmon and flaxseeds can curb inflammation, keeping milk ducts clear.

Some breastfeeding mothers find certain foods trigger plugged ducts, warranting the need for a food diary to identify potential culprits. Common triggers include dairy, caffeine, and spicy foods. Experimenting with elimination diets can help pinpoint problematic foods and alleviate symptoms.

Supplementation can also aid in preventing plugged ducts. Lecithin, a natural emulsifier, facilitates fat breakdown, promoting unhindered milk flow through ducts.

Adding a lecithin supplement to your regimen can prevent blockages and reduce the likelihood of plugged ducts. Additionally, vitamin E, an antioxidant, combats inflammation and supports healthy milk production, further reducing the risk of obstruction.

Before incorporating supplements, consult your healthcare provider, especially if pregnant or breastfeeding, to ensure safety and proper dosage.

Beyond dietary modifications and supplementation, optimizing breastfeeding techniques is crucial. Ensuring proper latch during feedings prevents incomplete drainage, minimizing blockage risk. Seeking assistance from a lactation consultant can refine breastfeeding techniques for optimal results.

Varying breastfeeding positions throughout the day ensures comprehensive breast emptying during feedings, mitigating blockage risk. Experiment with positions like the football hold or side-lying position to find what works best for you and your baby.

In conclusion, while breastfeeding presents its challenges, plugged ducts need not be one of them. By prioritizing hydration, maintaining a balanced diet, considering supplements, and optimizing breastfeeding techniques, nursing mothers can minimize the risk of plugged ducts, fostering a positive breastfeeding experience for both mother and baby.

Avoiding tight clothing and bras is essential to prevent pressure on the breasts, which can impede milk flow. Instead, opt for loose, comfortable attire that facilitates easy access during feedings. Additionally, incorporating breast massage before and during feedings can stimulate milk flow and deter blockages.

In the event of a plugged duct, several home remedies can aid in clearing it. Applying warm compresses to the affected area reduces inflammation and encourages milk flow.

Gentle massaging of the lump towards the nipple during feedings can also help dislodge the blockage. However, if the plugged duct persists beyond a day or two, or if symptoms of infection like fever arise, seeking medical attention is imperative.

In summary, while plugged ducts pose challenges for breastfeeding mothers, dietary adjustments and supplements can serve as preventative measures. Ensuring hydration, maintaining a balanced diet, and supplementing with substances like lecithin and vitamin E contribute to clear milk ducts and minimize blockage risk.

Coupled with sound breastfeeding techniques, avoiding constrictive clothing, and consulting with a lactation consultant as needed, these strategies promote a seamless breastfeeding journey for both mother and baby.

The Emotional Impact of Plugged Milk Ducts

Becoming a new mom is filled with joy and fulfillment, yet it also brings forth its set of obstacles. One such challenge that many new mothers encounter is dealing with plugged milk ducts.

This discomforting condition arises when a milk duct becomes obstructed, causing milk to accumulate and form a firm lump in the breast. Apart from the physical pain, plugged milk ducts can profoundly affect a new mother's emotional well-being.

The emotional toll of plugged milk ducts can be substantial, as it complicates breastfeeding, a vital aspect of bonding with the newborn. New moms often find themselves grappling with feelings of frustration, overwhelm, and even guilt when faced with difficulties in breastfeeding. Such emotions can breed a sense of inadequacy, triggering heightened levels of stress and anxiety.

Moreover, plugged milk ducts can exert a detrimental impact on a new mom's mental health.

The discomfort may hinder the bonding process with the baby and diminish the ability to relish the early stages of motherhood. Consequently, feelings of isolation, loneliness, and intensified depression and anxiety may ensue.

Thankfully, there exist coping mechanisms that new mothers can employ to navigate the emotional strain of dealing with plugged milk ducts. These strategies empower them to regain a sense of control amidst the challenges they face, while offering support and resources to help weather this trying period.

Foremost among these coping strategies is seeking support from healthcare professionals, lactation consultants, and fellow mothers who have confronted similar hurdles. Their insights, guidance, and empathy can serve as invaluable pillars of strength, alleviating the sense of isolation and providing practical assistance.

Equally crucial is the imperative for new mothers to prioritize their physical and emotional well-being during this period. This entails ensuring ample rest, maintaining a nourishing diet, staying hydrated, and engaging in activities that foster relaxation and stress relief.

By nurturing themselves, new moms cultivate resilience, enabling them to better navigate the challenges posed by plugged milk ducts.

Furthermore, practicing self-compassion and self-care is paramount for new moms grappling with plugged milk ducts. Acknowledging their efforts and embracing imperfection fosters a sense of confidence and diminishes feelings of guilt and self-doubt.

In addition to seeking support and nurturing oneself, employing relaxation techniques can aid in managing the emotional impact of plugged milk ducts. Activities like deep breathing exercises, meditation, yoga, and mindfulness practices offer solace, easing stress and fostering emotional equilibrium.

Ultimately, new moms should remember that plugged milk ducts are a common and treatable occurrence, and that seeking help and practicing self-care are vital steps toward managing the emotional strain associated with them. By drawing upon these coping strategies, new mothers can find solace amidst the challenges and relish the precious moments of motherhood.

In summary, while plugged milk ducts can bring about significant emotional challenges for new moms, there are effective coping strategies to navigate this condition.

By reaching out for support, prioritizing self-care, and embracing relaxation techniques, new mothers can reclaim a sense of empowerment and resilience, enabling them to cherish the early stages of motherhood more fully.

Remember, you're not alone in this journey, and there are numerous resources and supportive networks ready to assist you through this trying period.

Balancing Work and Breastfeeding

Juggling work responsibilities with breastfeeding presents a unique challenge for many mothers, often leading to the development of plugged ducts due to the demands of pumping breast milk while on the job.

Plugged ducts occur when milk ducts in the breast become obstructed, resulting in discomfort, swelling, and potential infection.

To prevent plugged ducts while on the move, meticulous planning and attention to detail are essential. Here are some strategies to help navigate this common breastfeeding issue:

1. Stay hydrated: Maintaining proper hydration is paramount in warding off plugged ducts. Ensure you drink an ample amount of water throughout the day, particularly during work hours. Adequate hydration helps maintain milk consistency, reducing the likelihood of duct blockages.

2. Stick to a pumping schedule: Establishing a consistent pumping routine while at work is crucial to prevent engorgement and plugged ducts. Aim to pump every 2-3 hours to ensure complete breast emptying, mitigating the risk of milk accumulation and subsequent blockages.

3. Invest in a quality breast pump: Choosing a reliable breast pump designed for frequent and efficient pumping can significantly reduce the risk of plugged ducts. Opt for a model optimized for regular use, and consider portability for convenience at work or while traveling.

4. Incorporate breast massage during pumping: During pumping sessions, gentle breast massage can promote milk flow and discourage blockages. Employ circular motions and light pressure to dislodge potential clogs within the milk ducts.

   This practice also aids in maintaining milk supply and preventing engorgement.

5. Prioritize relaxation breaks: Stress management is essential, as heightened stress levels can contribute to plugged ducts. Schedule regular breaks throughout the day to unwind and destress. Find a quiet space to pump where you can relax and concentrate on your breastfeeding session. Engage in deep breathing exercises and consciously release muscle tension to prevent blockages from forming.

By implementing these proactive measures, mothers can better navigate the challenges of balancing work commitments with breastfeeding, minimizing the risk of plugged ducts and promoting a smoother breastfeeding experience overall.

1. Wear comfortable and supportive clothing:

Wearing comfortable and supportive clothing while breastfeeding can help to prevent plugged ducts. Avoid tight bras or clothing that puts pressure on your breasts, as this can impede milk flow and lead to blockages. Opt for loose-fitting tops and nursing bras that provide proper support without constricting your breasts.

2. Prioritize hygiene: Maintaining cleanliness with your breast pump and accessories is crucial for preventing plugged ducts and potential infection.

3. Before each pumping session, wash your hands thoroughly, and diligently sanitize your pump parts afterward. Properly store your pump in a clean, dry environment to inhibit bacterial growth and safeguard against disruptions in milk flow.

4. Embrace heat therapy: Incorporating heat therapy into your pumping routine can effectively open up milk ducts and deter blockages. Before pumping, apply a warm compress or indulge in a warm shower to stimulate milk flow and thwart plugged ducts. Post-pumping, heat therapy can alleviate any discomfort or pain experienced.

5. Be vigilant for signs of plugged ducts: Familiarize yourself with the indicators of plugged ducts to address them promptly. Redness, swelling, or pain in the breast may signify a blocked duct. Employ gentle massage and heat application to alleviate blockages. Persistent

symptoms warrant consultation with your healthcare provider for further evaluation.

6. Consult a lactation consultant for support: Should you encounter difficulties in preventing plugged ducts while managing work and breastfeeding, seek assistance from a lactation consultant.

7. These professionals offer tailored advice and support to navigate breastfeeding challenges, ensuring a successful breastfeeding journey.

In summary, managing the balance between work and breastfeeding demands attention and planning to avoid plugged ducts while on the move.

Prioritize cleanliness, integrate heat therapy, remain vigilant for signs of blockages, and seek professional support as needed. With these proactive measures, you can navigate the complexities of breastfeeding while working and minimize the occurrence of plugged ducts.

Chapter5: The Connection Between Mastitis and Plugged Milk Ducts

Mastitis and plugged milk ducts are prevalent challenges for breastfeeding women, each impacting the breastfeeding journey distinctly. Understanding their correlation is pivotal for effective management and prevention strategies.

Mastitis signifies inflammation of breast tissue, often due to bacterial infection, presenting symptoms like redness, swelling, pain, and warmth. Additionally, flu-like symptoms such as fever and body aches may manifest. Seeking medical attention promptly upon suspicion of mastitis is crucial to avert potential complications.

Plugged milk ducts, conversely, emerge when milk removal from the breast is inefficient, resulting in duct blockage, accompanied by pain, swelling, and lump formation. Left untreated, plugged ducts can escalate to mastitis if infection sets in.

The nexus between mastitis and plugged milk ducts underscores the progression from the latter to the former. Inadequate milk removal fosters milk stagnation, rendering it susceptible to bacterial proliferation, culminating in inflammation and infection—manifestations characteristic of mastitis. Timely resolution of plugged ducts is hence imperative to forestall mastitis onset.

Various factors contribute to plugged ducts and mastitis development:

- Suboptimal latching: Incorrect latching impedes effective breast emptying, predisposing to plugged ducts.

- Engorgement: Breast engorgement obstructs milk flow, fostering plugged duct formation.

- Infrequent feedings: Sporadic feedings encourage milk stasis, fostering plugged ducts.

- Breast pressure: Ill-fitting bras or constrictive attire exert pressure on the breast, provoking duct blockage.
- Stress and fatigue: Weakened immunity due to stress and fatigue heightens susceptibility to infection.

Prevention of plugged ducts and mastitis necessitates ensuring optimal breast emptying and nurturing breast health.

Here are essential practices to prevent plugged milk ducts and mastitis:

- **Ensuring proper latch**: Correct positioning and latching facilitate effective breast emptying during feedings.

- **Nursing frequently**: On-demand nursing and complete breast emptying during each feeding help avert engorgement and plugged ducts.

- **Using varied nursing positions**: Altering nursing positions ensures thorough breast emptying across all areas.

- **Avoiding breast pressure**: Opting for loose-fitting attire and well-fitted bras minimizes pressure on the breast.

- **Managing stress and fatigue**: Reducing stress levels and obtaining sufficient rest supports overall breast health.

In case of plugged milk ducts, these steps can help resolve them and prevent mastitis:

- **Frequent nursing**: Nursing on demand and ensuring complete emptying of the affected breast at each feeding helps clear plugged ducts.

- **Warm compresses**: Application of warm compresses promotes milk flow and alleviates pain.

- **Breast massage**: Gently massaging the affected breast aids in dislodging the blockage and stimulating milk flow.

- **Varied nursing positions**: Changing nursing positions ensures effective emptying of the affected breast area.

- **Over-the-counter pain relievers**: Ibuprofen and similar medications can help manage pain and inflammation.

If mastitis arises, prompt medical attention is crucial. Treatment typically involves antibiotics to eradicate the infection and measures to alleviate pain and inflammation. Continuing breastfeeding is usually advised as it aids in resolving the infection and preventing further complications.

In conclusion, understanding the link between mastitis and plugged milk ducts is vital for prevention and treatment. By adhering to practices that ensure proper breast emptying, managing stress levels, and promptly addressing any issues, women can support their breastfeeding journey and maintain optimal breast health.

Navigating the Challenges of Breastfeeding with Plugged Ducts

Breastfeeding is a natural and fulfilling experience, yet it can present mothers with various hurdles. Among these challenges, plugged ducts stand out as a common issue, complicating the breastfeeding journey. In this discussion, we'll delve into the complexities of breastfeeding amidst plugged ducts, offering insights and practical advice from a maternal perspective.

Understanding Plugged Ducts:

Plugged ducts manifest when a milk duct in the breast becomes obstructed, impeding the smooth flow of milk. This obstruction induces pain, swelling, and redness in the affected breast. Several factors contribute to plugged ducts, including:

- Incorrect latching or positioning during breastfeeding.
- Wearing tight or constrictive attire.
- Irregular breastfeeding or pumping schedules.
- Elevated stress levels or fatigue.
- Underlying illness or infection.

The buildup of milk behind the blockage exacerbates discomfort for the mother, potentially escalating into mastitis—an agonizing breast infection—if untreated.

Strategies for Navigating Breastfeeding Challenges:

Breastfeeding while contending with plugged ducts can be a taxing ordeal for mothers. Nonetheless, employing certain strategies can alleviate symptoms and thwart future blockages.

Here are actionable tips for maneuvering through breastfeeding with plugged ducts:

1. Prioritize Proper Latching and Positioning:

Improper latching and positioning rank among the primary culprits behind plugged ducts. Ensuring that your baby latches correctly and is positioned optimally can significantly reduce the likelihood of blockages. Seek assistance from a lactation consultant if you frequently encounter plugged ducts, ensuring both you and your baby are breastfeeding effectively.

1. Breastfeed Regularly and Thoroughly

Consistent and thorough breastfeeding sessions play a vital role in preventing the formation of plugged ducts. Ensure you breastfeed your baby on demand and allow them to fully empty each breast before switching sides. If your baby isn't nursing effectively, consider incorporating a breast pump to aid in completely emptying your breasts.

2. Embrace Heat Therapy and Massage

Utilizing heat on the affected breast can effectively loosen the blockage and enhance milk flow. You can apply warmth through a warm compress, heating pad, or by indulging in a warm shower to alleviate discomfort. Additionally, gentle massage of the affected breast can help disintegrate the blockage and stimulate milk flow.

3. Employ Cold Therapy

Post-nursing or pumping, applying a cold compress to the affected breast can effectively reduce swelling and inflammation. Cold compresses not only offer numbing relief but also alleviate pain and discomfort.

4. Prioritize Hydration and Rest

Maintaining optimal hydration levels and ensuring sufficient rest are crucial in sustaining a healthy milk supply and thwarting plugged ducts. Make it a point to drink ample water throughout the day and take adequate breaks to rejuvenate and unwind.

5. Opt for Comfortable Attire

Avoiding tight or constrictive clothing is essential as it can exert unnecessary pressure on the breasts, leading to plugged ducts. Opt for loose-fitting, breathable attire that facilitates proper airflow and unrestricted movement. Steer clear of underwire bras and snug sports bras that may impede breast health.

6. Address Stress and Fatigue

Managing stress levels and combating fatigue are paramount to maintaining optimal milk production and minimizing the risk of plugged ducts. Prioritize self-care by effectively managing stress, ensuring adequate sleep, and seeking support from your support network. Incorporate relaxation techniques such as deep breathing exercises, meditation, or yoga to foster a serene breastfeeding experience.

1. Reach Out for Support and Advice

When facing challenges like plugged ducts during breastfeeding, it's essential not to hesitate in seeking support and guidance. Whether it's from a lactation consultant, healthcare provider, or a breastfeeding support group, reaching out to professionals and fellow mothers can provide valuable advice, encouragement, and resources to help navigate these hurdles effectively.

A Mother's Perspective on Breastfeeding with Plugged Ducts

Breastfeeding while dealing with plugged ducts can present significant challenges and frustrations for mothers. To delve into the realities of this experience, we had a conversation with Sarah, a mother of two who encountered plugged ducts while nursing her children.

Sarah candidly shared her journey with plugged ducts and the strategies she employed to manage this common breastfeeding complication.

Reflecting on her first encounter with plugged ducts shortly after her first child's birth, Sarah recounted, "I had heard about plugged ducts before, but I never anticipated experiencing it myself. The pain and discomfort were overwhelming, and I felt lost."

Seeking assistance from a lactation consultant proved instrumental for Sarah. "The consultant guided me through techniques like applying heat and gentle massage to the affected breast," she explained.

How to Clear Plugged Milk Ducts Quickly and Effectively

Experiencing a plugged milk duct can be a challenging ordeal for breastfeeding mothers, causing pain and frustration. This condition arises when one of the milk ducts in the breast becomes obstructed, hindering the smooth flow of milk.

Consequently, this blockage leads to milk buildup, swelling, and inflammation in the affected breast. If left unaddressed, a plugged milk duct can escalate into mastitis, a more severe condition characterized by flu-like symptoms and potentially requiring medical intervention.

Thankfully, there are several effective methods to promptly and efficiently clear plugged milk ducts. By adhering to these strategies, you can alleviate discomfort and stave off further complications.

1. Prioritize Frequent and Effective Nursing

A crucial step in clearing a plugged milk duct is frequent and efficient nursing. Ensure your baby is latching correctly and thoroughly emptying the breast during each feeding session. This helps prevent milk accumulation in the ducts and minimizes the risk of blockages.

If you detect a plugged duct, increase nursing sessions on the affected side. Position your baby in a way that their chin faces the blocked duct, facilitating its clearance. Additionally, gentle massage of the affected breast during nursing can aid in breaking up the blockage and enhancing milk flow.

2. Utilize Heat Therapy

Applying heat to the affected breast can mitigate inflammation and enhance milk flow. Employ warm compresses, heating pads, or indulge in a warm shower to administer heat to the blocked duct. Aim to apply heat for 10-15 minutes before nursing to soften the blockage and facilitate smoother milk flow.

1. Employ Gentle Breast Massage

Gently massaging the affected breast can effectively dislodge the blockage and enhance milk flow. Using your fingertips, apply circular motions around the blocked duct area. Alternatively, try softly squeezing the breast from its base towards the nipple to encourage the blockage's clearance.

2. Utilize a Breast Pump

When nursing on the affected side proves challenging for your baby or if you're unable to nurse frequently enough to resolve the blockage, employing a breast pump can be beneficial.

Pumping aids in alleviating engorgement and promoting milk flow within the obstructed duct. Opt for a comfortable and efficient breast pump, and consider pumping on the affected side post-nursing to aid in clearing the blockage.

3. Experiment with Various Nursing Positions

Exploring different nursing positions may facilitate the clearance of a plugged duct. Experiment with positions like the football hold or the side-lying posture to enhance milk flow and alleviate the blockage.

Continuously try different positions until discovering one that's both comfortable and effective for you and your baby.

4. Maintain Hydration and Proper Nutrition

Sustaining adequate hydration and nourishment is crucial for preserving a healthy milk supply and preventing blocked ducts. Ensure you consume ample water throughout the day and maintain a balanced diet rich in fruits, vegetables, and whole grains. Steer clear of caffeinated and alcoholic beverages, as they can lead to dehydration and impact your milk production.

1. Prioritize Rest

Rest is paramount for breastfeeding mothers, particularly when contending with a plugged milk duct. Ensure you allocate sufficient time for rest and incorporate breaks throughout the day to unwind and rejuvenate.

Nap whenever your baby does, and don't hesitate to seek assistance from loved ones if needed. Managing stress and fatigue is crucial in preventing and resolving blocked ducts, so prioritize self-care to maintain your well-being.

2. Employ Cold Compresses

Besides utilizing heat therapy on the affected breast, integrating cold compresses can aid in reducing inflammation and alleviating discomfort.

Employ a cold pack, a packet of frozen vegetables, or even a chilled cabbage leaf to apply cold to the affected area. Alternating between heat and cold compresses can enhance milk flow and diminish discomfort effectively.

3. Consider Over-the-Counter Pain Relievers

Should you experience pain and discomfort due to a plugged milk duct, consider taking over-the-counter pain relievers like ibuprofen or acetaminophen to alleviate symptoms.

Adhere to the recommended dosage outlined on the medication packaging, and consult with your healthcare provider if you have any queries or concerns.

4. Seek Guidance from a Lactation Consultant

If you encounter challenges in clearing a plugged milk duct or experience recurrent blockages, consulting with a lactation consultant can offer invaluable assistance.

A lactation consultant can furnish personalized guidance and support to refine your breastfeeding technique, mitigate future blockages, and ensure your baby receives adequate nourishment. They can also help troubleshoot any nursing difficulties you may encounter and provide additional resources and assistance.

In summary, while a plugged milk duct may pose challenges for breastfeeding mothers, employing various strategies can effectively resolve blockages. By prioritizing rest, utilizing cold compresses, considering pain relievers, and seeking guidance from a lactation consultant, you can navigate this obstacle and sustain a fulfilling breastfeeding journey.

Chapter6: The Benefits of Lecithin Supplements in Preventing Plugged Ducts

Lecithin supplements have gained popularity in recent years for their potential benefits in preventing plugged ducts, especially in breastfeeding mothers.

Plugged ducts can be a painful and frustrating experience for many women, and finding ways to prevent them can be crucial for maintaining breastfeeding success.

In this article, we will explore the benefits of lecithin supplements in preventing plugged ducts and how they can be a valuable addition to a breastfeeding mother's routine.

What are Plugged Ducts?

Plugged ducts occur when a milk duct in the breast becomes blocked, preventing the flow of milk. This blockage can cause pain, swelling, and inflammation in the affected breast, making it difficult for milk to be expressed.

Plugged ducts are a common issue for breastfeeding mothers, and they can be caused by a variety of factors, including:

- Improper latch or positioning during breastfeeding
- Wearing tight-fitting bras or clothing that puts pressure on the breasts
- Infrequent or irregular breastfeeding or pumping
- Stress or fatigue
- Dehydration
- Mastitis (a bacterial infection of the breast tissue)

Plugged ducts can be uncomfortable and can interfere with a mother's ability to breastfeed effectively. In severe cases, they can lead to mastitis, a more serious condition that requires medical treatment.

Finding ways to prevent plugged ducts is essential for maintaining breastfeeding success and ensuring the health and well-being of both mother and baby.

How Lecithin Supplements Can Help

Lecithin is a natural substance found in many foods, including egg yolks, soybeans, and organ meats. It is a complex mixture of phospholipids that are essential for the structure and function of cell membranes.

Lecithin supplements are derived from soybeans and are available in capsule or granule form. They are commonly used as a dietary supplement to support brain health, liver function, and cholesterol levels.

Lecithin supplements have also been found to be beneficial in preventing plugged ducts in breastfeeding mothers. The exact mechanism by which lecithin helps prevent plugged ducts is not fully understood, but it is believed to be related to its ability to reduce the viscosity of breast milk.

By making the milk less thick and sticky, lecithin can help prevent blockages in the milk ducts and promote better milk flow.

In a study published in the Journal of Human Lactation, researchers found that lecithin supplements were effective in reducing the frequency of plugged ducts in breastfeeding mothers.

The study involved 120 women who were randomly assigned to take either lecithin supplements or a placebo for six weeks. The results showed that women who took lecithin supplements had a significantly lower incidence of plugged ducts compared to those who took the placebo.

In addition to preventing plugged ducts, lecithin supplements may also help improve the quality of breast milk. Lecithin is a source of choline, a nutrient that is important for brain development and function. By increasing the
choline content of breast milk, lecithin supplements may provide additional benefits for the baby's cognitive development and overall health.

How to Use Lecithin Supplements

If you are a breastfeeding mother who is experiencing plugged ducts or are at risk for developing them, adding lecithin supplements to your daily routine may be beneficial.

Lecithin supplements are generally safe and well- tolerated, but it is important to consult with your healthcare provider before starting any new supplement regimen.

The recommended dosage of lecithin supplements for preventing plugged ducts is typically 1,200-1,600 milligrams per day, divided into three or four doses. It is best to take lecithin supplements with meals to enhance absorption and minimize gastrointestinal side effects.

 It may take several weeks for the full benefits of lecithin supplements to be realized, so be patient and consistent with your supplementation routine.

In addition to taking lecithin supplements, there are several other steps you can take to prevent plugged ducts while breastfeeding:

- Ensure proper latch and positioning during breastfeeding
- Feed your baby frequently and on demand
- Avoid wearing tight-fitting bras or clothing
- Stay hydrated and well-nourished
- Get plenty of rest and manage stress levels

By incorporating lecithin supplements into your daily routine and following these preventive measures, you can reduce your risk of developing plugged ducts and enjoy a more comfortable and successful breastfeeding experience.

Plugged ducts are a common and frustrating issue for many breastfeeding mothers, but they can be effectively prevented with the help of lecithin supplements.

By reducing the viscosity of breast milk and promoting better milk flow, lecithin supplements can help prevent blockages in the milk ducts and improve the quality of breast milk.

Understanding the Role of Hormones in Plugged Milk Ducts

Plugged milk ducts pose a common challenge for many breastfeeding mothers, often causing pain and frustration.

However, understanding the hormonal dynamics underlying this issue can empower you to effectively manage and prevent it.

Hormones, such as prolactin and oxytocin, play pivotal roles in lactation and milk production. Prolactin triggers milk production in the mammary glands upon childbirth, sustaining it throughout breastfeeding. Concurrently, oxytocin facilitates milk flow from the glands to the nipple during nursing, facilitating the feeding process.

Plugged milk ducts ensue when milk remains inadequately drained from the breast, owing to factors like improper latch, infrequent nursing, or constrictive attire. Accumulation of milk within the ducts leads to obstruction, causing inflammation, pain, and swelling.

Hormonal fluctuations further contribute to plugged ducts by potentially inducing milk oversupply, intensifying duct pressure, and compromising duct elasticity postpartum.

Understanding the hormonal influence on plugged milk ducts enables proactive prevention and management strategies. Ensuring effective milk removal during feeding sessions—via correct latch, on-demand feeding, and diverse nursing positions—can mitigate the risk of blockages.

Should plugged ducts manifest, applying heat to the affected area before nursing or pumping can alleviate symptoms by easing blockage and enhancing milk flow. Additionally, gentle massage during feeding or pumping aids in dislodging the blockage and promoting milk expulsion.

In some instances, healthcare providers may recommend over-the-counter pain relievers or anti-inflammatory drugs to alleviate associated discomfort and inflammation. However, consulting a healthcare professional before medication intake while breastfeeding is crucial to ensure safety for both mother and baby.

If you find yourself grappling with recurring plugged ducts, seeking guidance from a lactation consultant or healthcare provider can offer valuable insights. They can assist in identifying any underlying factors contributing to the issue and offer strategies to mitigate future occurrences.

In summary, hormones wield considerable influence over plugged milk ducts' development. Empowering yourself with knowledge about their role in lactation and milk production enables proactive measures to address and navigate this prevalent challenge.

Should plugged ducts arise, reaching out to a healthcare provider or lactation consultant ensures optimal health and comfort for both you and your baby throughout the breastfeeding voyage.

The Link Between Engorgement and Plugged Ducts: How to Find Relief

Engorgement and plugged ducts are common issues that many breastfeeding mothers face. While they are often related, they can also occur independently of each other.

Understanding the link between engorgement and plugged ducts can help mothers find relief and continue breastfeeding successfully.

Engorgement occurs when the breasts become overly full of milk. This can happen for a variety of reasons, such as when a mother's milk first comes in after giving birth, when a baby suddenly nurses less frequently, or when a mother skips feedings or pumping sessions.

Engorgement can be uncomfortable and even painful, as the breasts become swollen, hard, and sometimes hot to the touch.

Plugged ducts, on the other hand, occur when a milk duct becomes blocked.

This blockage can be caused by a variety of factors, including pressure on the breast from tight clothing or a poorly fitting bra, infrequent feedings or pumping sessions, or even stress or fatigue.

Plugged ducts can be painful and can lead to more serious issues if not addressed promptly.

The link between engorgement and plugged ducts is that engorgement can lead to plugged ducts. When the breasts are overly full of milk, it can put pressure on the milk ducts and make them more susceptible to becoming blocked.

This is why it is important for mothers to address engorgement promptly to prevent plugged ducts from occurring.

Finding relief from engorgement and plugged ducts involves a combination of strategies, including frequent feedings or pumping sessions, proper breast care, and sometimes medication or other treatments. Here are some tips for finding relief from engorgement and plugged ducts:

1.   Nurse frequently: The best way to prevent and relieve engorgement and plugged ducts is to nurse your baby frequently. This helps to empty the breasts regularly and prevent them from becoming overly full. If your baby is not nursing frequently enough, try to pump to relieve the pressure and prevent blockages.

2.   Use proper breastfeeding techniques: Make sure your baby is latched on correctly and nursing effectively. Poor latch can lead to inefficient milk removal and increase the risk of engorgement and plugged ducts. If you are having trouble with latching, seek help from a lactation consultant or breastfeeding support group.

3.   Apply heat: Applying heat to the affected breast can help to relieve engorgement and plugged ducts. You can use a warm compress, a heating pad, or even take a warm shower to help soften the breast tissue and promote milk flow.

4.   Massage the breast: Gently massaging the affected breast can help to break up any blockages and promote milk flow. You can use your fingers to massage in a circular motion towards the nipple, or use a breast massage tool to help release any trapped milk.

5.   Use cold packs: After nursing or pumping, you can apply cold packs to the breasts to help reduce swelling and inflammation. This can help to relieve pain and discomfort associated with engorgement and plugged ducts.

6.   Stay hydrated and well-nourished: Make sure you are drinking plenty of water and eating a balanced diet to support your milk supply and overall breastfeeding health. Dehydration and poor nutrition can contribute to engorgement and plugged ducts, so it is important to take care of yourself.

7.   Get plenty of rest: Rest is important for breastfeeding mothers, as fatigue and stress can contribute to engorgement and plugged ducts. Make sure you are getting enough sleep and taking time to relax and recharge.

8.   Seek help if needed: If you are experiencing severe pain, fever, or other symptoms of infection, it is important to seek help from a healthcare provider. In some cases, antibiotics or other treatments may be necessary to address engorgement and plugged ducts.

Overall, the link between engorgement and plugged ducts is clear: engorgement can lead to blocked ducts, which can be painful and even lead to more serious issues if not addressed promptly.

By following the tips outlined above and seeking help if needed, breastfeeding mothers can find relief from engorgement and plugged ducts and continue to breastfeed successfully.

Remember, you are not alone in facing these challenges, and there is support available to help you navigate this journey.

Chapter7: Lifestyle Changes for Preventing Plugged Milk Ducts in the Long Term

Plugged milk ducts can be a painful and frustrating experience for breastfeeding mothers. They occur when milk flow is blocked in the ducts, leading to a build-up of milk and inflammation in the breast tissue.

This can cause discomfort, swelling, and even infection if not properly addressed.

While plugged milk ducts can happen to any breastfeeding mother, there are certain lifestyle changes that can help prevent them in the long term.

By incorporating these changes into your daily routine, you can reduce your risk of developing plugged milk ducts and ensure a smoother breastfeeding experience for both you and your baby.

1. Proper Breastfeeding Positioning

One of the most important factors in preventing plugged milk ducts is ensuring proper breastfeeding positioning. When your baby is latched on correctly and feeding effectively, it helps to prevent milk from backing up in the ducts and causing blockages.

Make sure your baby is latched on deeply and that their nose is aligned with your nipple. You should also switch sides frequently during feedings to ensure that all parts of your breast are being emptied regularly.

2. Emptying Your Breasts Fully

Another key to preventing plugged milk ducts is to ensure that your breasts are fully emptied during each feeding. If your baby is not feeding effectively or if you are not emptying your breasts completely, milk can back up in the ducts and lead to blockages. Make sure to nurse your baby on demand and to pump any excess milk if needed to ensure that your breasts are fully emptied after each feeding.

3. Avoiding Tight Clothing and Underwire Bras

Wearing tight clothing or underwire bras can put pressure on your breasts and restrict milk flow, leading to plugged milk ducts. Opt for loose-fitting, comfortable clothing and bras that provide proper support without constricting your breasts. You may also want to consider wearing a nursing bra that allows for easy access during feedings and pumping sessions.

4. Maintaining Proper Hygiene

Good hygiene is essential for preventing plugged milk ducts and other breast infections. Make sure to wash your hands before breastfeeding or pumping to prevent the spread of germs. You should also clean your breast pump and bottles regularly to avoid contamination.

If you notice any signs of infection, such as redness, swelling, or pain in your breasts, contact your healthcare provider for treatment.

5. Managing Stress Levels

Stress can have a negative impact on breastfeeding and can increase your risk of developing plugged milk ducts. Finding ways to manage stress, such as practicing relaxation techniques, getting enough sleep, and seeking support from loved ones, can help to reduce your risk of developing blockages.

Make time for self-care and prioritize your mental and emotional well-being to support a healthy breastfeeding experience.

6. Staying Hydrated and Eating a Balanced Diet

Proper hydration and nutrition are essential for maintaining milk supply and preventing plugged milk ducts. Make sure to drink plenty of water throughout the day to stay hydrated and support milk production.

Eating a balanced diet rich in fruits, vegetables, whole grains, and lean proteins can also help to keep your body healthy and functioning optimally. Avoiding excessive caffeine and alcohol consumption can also help to prevent dehydration and support breastfeeding.

7. Engaging in Regular Exercise

Regular exercise can help to improve circulation and prevent blockages in the milk ducts. Engaging in low- impact activities such as walking, swimming, or yoga can help to keep your body healthy and reduce your risk of developing plugged milk ducts.

Make sure to wear a supportive bra during exercise to prevent discomfort and strain on your breasts.

8. Using Warm Compresses and Massaging Your Breasts

If you are prone to plugged milk ducts, using warm compresses and massaging your breasts can help to prevent blockages and relieve discomfort. Applying a warm compress to your breasts before feedings can help to soften the milk and improve milk flow.

Massaging your breasts gently during feedings or pumping sessions can also help to break up any blockages and prevent them from forming.

9. Seeking Professional Help if Needed

If you are experiencing frequent plugged milk ducts despite making lifestyle changes, it may be helpful to seek professional help from a lactation consultant or healthcare provider.

They can provide personalized advice and support to help you address any underlying issues that may be contributing to your recurrent blockages. They may also recommend additional treatments, such as medication or physical therapy, to help prevent plugged milk ducts in the long term.

10. Being Patient and Persistent

Preventing plugged milk ducts requires patience and persistence. It may take time to find the right combination of lifestyle changes that work for you and your baby. Be patient with yourself and continue to make adjustments as needed to support a healthy breastfeeding experience.

Remember that every mother and baby are unique, and what works for one may not work for another. Stay positive and focused on your goal of preventing plugged milk ducts and providing the best possible care for your baby.

The Impact of Stress on Milk Production and Duct Health

Stress is a ubiquitous aspect of modern life that profoundly impacts our physical and mental well-being. However, its effects extend beyond these realms to influence milk production and duct health in lactating women.

This article delves into the intricate relationship between stress and breastfeeding, shedding light on how it can affect milk supply and duct health.

Breastfeeding, a natural phenomenon, boasts myriad benefits for both mother and baby. Yet, many women grapple with the challenge of low milk supply, a source of considerable stress and dismay.

Stress can disrupt the production of prolactin, the hormone pivotal for milk synthesis. Elevated stress prompts the release of cortisol, a stress hormone that hampers prolactin production, consequently diminishing milk supply.

Beyond its impact on milk production, stress exerts a deleterious effect on milk duct health. Milk ducts serve as conduits, transporting milk from the mammary glands to the nipples for infant consumption. Stress triggers the release of inflammatory markers, inciting inflammation and damage within the milk ducts.

This cascade of events precipitates blocked ducts, mastitis, and other breastfeeding complications.

Empirical evidence underscores the correlation between heightened stress levels and breastfeeding challenges, including reduced milk supply and duct issues.

A study featured in the journal Breastfeeding Medicine revealed that women experiencing elevated stress levels exhibited diminished milk production and were more prone to encountering breastfeeding hurdles compared to their less stressed counterparts.

To enhance milk production and duct health while breastfeeding, women can employ various strategies aimed at stress reduction and overall well-being. Prioritizing self-care and relaxation stands as a pivotal step. This entails carving out time for oneself, practicing mindfulness and meditation, ensuring sufficient sleep, and indulging in activities that promote joy and tranquility.

Equally crucial is the support garnered from family, friends, and healthcare providers, as it significantly influences breastfeeding outcomes. Women who feel bolstered and empowered are more likely to navigate breastfeeding challenges with resilience and vigor.

Seeking guidance from lactation consultants or participating in breastfeeding support groups offers invaluable assistance for those encountering hurdles.

Adopting a healthy lifestyle further contributes to stress mitigation and supports milk production and duct health. Maintaining a balanced diet, staying adequately hydrated, and engaging in regular exercise foster overall well-being, thereby fostering breastfeeding success.

Abstaining from alcohol, caffeine, and tobacco likewise fosters optimal milk production and duct health.

It's vital for women to recognize that breastfeeding is a natural process that unfolds with patience, practice, and support. Should stress or breastfeeding difficulties arise, seeking assistance is encouraged.

Whether from a healthcare provider, lactation consultant, or breastfeeding support group, valuable resources and guidance are available to help surmount obstacles and nurture a fulfilling breastfeeding journey.

In essence, stress can significantly impact milk production and duct health in lactating women. By prioritizing self-care, seeking support, and embracing a healthy lifestyle, women can mitigate stress and foster breastfeeding success.

Remember, breastfeeding is a journey marked by patience and support, and seeking assistance when needed ensures a positive experience for both mother and baby.

The Connection Between Breastfeeding Positions and Plugged Ducts

Breastfeeding is a beautiful and natural way for mothers to nourish their babies. However, it can also come with its challenges, one of which is plugged ducts.

Plugged ducts occur when milk ducts in the breast become blocked, leading to discomfort, pain, and potentially even infection. While there are many factors that can contribute to plugged ducts, one important factor to consider is the breastfeeding position.

Breastfeeding positions play a crucial role in ensuring proper milk flow and preventing plugged ducts.

The way a mother positions her baby at the breast can impact how effectively the milk is drained from the breast, which in turn can affect the likelihood of developing plugged ducts.

In this article, we will explore the connection between breastfeeding positions and plugged ducts, and provide tips on how to prevent and treat this common breastfeeding issue.

Different breastfeeding positions can affect milk flow and drainage in the breast. Some positions may put more pressure on certain areas of the breast, leading to poor drainage and potential blockages.

For example, the football hold position, where the baby is held under the arm like a football, can sometimes put pressure on the ducts along the sides of the breast, making them more prone to becoming blocked.

On the other hand, the cradle hold position, where the baby is held in the crook of the mother's arm, may provide more even pressure on the breast and promote better milk flow.

Another factor to consider is the angle at which the baby latches onto the breast. A shallow latch can compress the ducts and prevent milk from flowing freely, increasing the risk of plugged ducts.

It is important for mothers to ensure that their baby has a deep latch, with the baby's mouth covering a large portion of the areola.

This helps to ensure that the milk ducts are properly drained during feeding, reducing the likelihood of blockages.

In addition to the breastfeeding position and latch, other factors can also contribute to plugged ducts. These include infrequent feedings, tight clothing or bras that put pressure on the breasts, and improper breast pump use.

It is important for mothers to be mindful of these factors and take steps to prevent plugged ducts from occurring.

If a mother does develop a plugged duct, there are several steps she can take to help resolve the issue. One effective method is to apply warm compresses to the affected area and gently massage the breast to help loosen the blockage.

It is also important for the mother to continue breastfeeding frequently, as emptying the breast regularly can help to clear the blockage.

In some cases, a healthcare provider may recommend taking over-the- counter pain relievers or using a prescription medication to help reduce inflammation and pain associated with plugged ducts.

In conclusion, breastfeeding positions play a crucial role in preventing plugged ducts and ensuring proper milk flow.

Mothers should be mindful of their breastfeeding position and latch, as well as other factors that can contribute to plugged ducts. By taking steps to promote good milk drainage and seeking help if a plugged duct does occur, mothers can continue to breastfeed successfully and provide their babies with the nourishment they need.

Chapter8: The Role of Latching Techniques in Preventing Plugged Milk Ducts

Breastfeeding is a natural and beautiful process that provides numerous benefits for both the mother and the baby. However, it can also come with its fair share of challenges, one of which is plugged milk ducts.

Plugged milk ducts occur when the milk flow in the breast is blocked, leading to pain, swelling, and potential infection. One of the key factors in preventing plugged milk ducts is the proper latching technique.

Latching is the way in which the baby attaches to the breast to feed. A good latch is crucial for effective breastfeeding, as it ensures that the baby is able to effectively remove milk from the breast.

When a baby latches on correctly, they are able to create a vacuum that allows them to suckle efficiently. This not only ensures that the baby is getting enough milk, but it also helps to prevent plugged milk ducts.

There are several key elements to achieving a good latch. Firstly, the baby should be positioned correctly at the breast. This means that the baby's mouth should be wide open, with their lips flanged outwards.

The baby's chin should be pressed into the breast, and their nose should be free from obstruction. The baby should also have a good mouthful of breast tissue in their mouth, with the nipple pointing towards the roof of their mouth.

In addition to positioning, it is important to ensure that the baby is latching on correctly. This means that the baby should have a deep latch, with their mouth covering as much of the areola as possible.

The baby's tongue should be extended over the lower gum, and their lips should be flanged outwards. A good latch should not be painful for the mother, and the baby should be able to suckle effectively.

When a baby latches on incorrectly, it can lead to a shallow latch. This means that the baby is not able to effectively remove milk from the breast, which can lead to plugged milk ducts.

A shallow latch can also cause pain and discomfort for the mother, as the baby may be sucking on the nipple rather than the areola. This can lead to nipple damage and potential infection.

There are several signs that indicate a shallow latch. These include pain during feeding, nipple damage, and a clicking sound while the baby is feeding.

If a mother is experiencing any of these symptoms, it is important to seek help from a lactation consultant or healthcare provider to correct the latch and prevent plugged milk ducts.

In addition to proper latching technique, there are several other factors that can help to prevent plugged milk ducts. One of the most important factors is frequent feeding.

By feeding the baby frequently, the mother is able to ensure that the milk is flowing effectively and that the breasts are being emptied regularly. This can help to prevent milk from becoming stagnant in the ducts and causing a blockage.

It is also important for the mother to ensure that she is taking care of her breasts properly.

This includes wearing a supportive bra, avoiding tight clothing that can restrict milk flow, and using warm compresses or massaging the breasts to help prevent plugged ducts.

 It is also important for the mother to stay hydrated and well-nourished, as this can help to ensure that the milk supply is adequate and that the breasts are functioning properly.

In some cases, despite taking all the necessary precautions, a mother may still develop plugged milk ducts. If this occurs, it is important for the mother to seek help from a healthcare provider.

They may recommend techniques such as warm compresses, massage, and frequent feeding to help clear the blockage. In some cases, a healthcare provider may also prescribe medication to help reduce inflammation and pain.

Overall, the role of latching techniques in preventing plugged milk ducts is crucial. By ensuring that the baby is latching on correctly, the mother can help to ensure that the milk is flowing effectively and that the breasts are being emptied regularly.

 This can help to prevent plugged milk ducts and ensure a successful breastfeeding relationship between the mother and baby.

In conclusion, breastfeeding is a beautiful and natural process that provides numerous benefits for both the mother and the baby.

However, it can also come with its fair share of challenges, one of which is plugged milk ducts. By focusing on proper latching techniques, frequent feeding, and taking care of the breasts, mothers can help to prevent plugged milk ducts and ensure a successful breastfeeding relationship.

If a mother does develop plugged milk ducts, it is important to seek help from a healthcare provider to address the issue promptly.

With the right support and guidance, mothers can overcome plugged milk ducts and continue to enjoy the many benefits of breastfeeding.

The Benefits of Breastfeeding on Demand

Breastfeeding is a natural and essential way to nourish a baby, providing them with all the nutrients they need to grow and develop.

One of the key benefits of breastfeeding on demand is its ability to prevent plugged ducts, a common issue that can arise when breastfeeding.

In this article, we will explore the benefits of breastfeeding on demand in preventing plugged ducts and how it can help both mother and baby.

Plugged ducts occur when milk ducts in the breast become blocked, leading to a build-up of milk and causing discomfort and pain for the mother.

This can happen for a variety of reasons, such as infrequent breastfeeding, poor latch, or pressure on the breasts. When a duct becomes blocked, it can lead to inflammation and infection, known as mastitis, which can be a serious condition requiring medical attention.

Breastfeeding on demand, also known as responsive feeding, involves feeding the baby whenever they show signs of hunger, rather than following a strict feeding schedule.

This approach allows the baby to regulate their own intake and ensures they are getting enough milk to meet their needs. By breastfeeding on demand, the mother is also able to empty her breasts regularly, which helps to prevent blocked ducts from occurring.

One of the key benefits of breastfeeding on demand in preventing plugged ducts is that it helps to maintain a good milk supply.

When the breasts are emptied regularly, the body receives signals to produce more milk, ensuring that the baby is adequately nourished. This can help to prevent engorgement, a common precursor to plugged ducts, as well as ensuring that the baby is getting enough milk to support their growth and development.

Another benefit of breastfeeding on demand is that it allows for better milk flow. When a baby is allowed to feed whenever they are hungry, they are more likely to empty the breast fully, ensuring that the milk ducts are clear and free-flowing.

 This can help to prevent blocked ducts from occurring, as well as reducing the risk of mastitis and other complications.

Breastfeeding on demand also helps to promote good latch and positioning, which are essential for effective breastfeeding.

When a baby is allowed to feed whenever they are hungry, they are more likely to latch on correctly and nurse effectively. This can help to prevent nipple pain and damage, as well as ensuring that the baby is able to get enough milk during each feeding session.

In addition to preventing plugged ducts, breastfeeding on demand has a number of other benefits for both mother and baby.

For the mother, breastfeeding on demand can help to promote bonding with the baby, as well as providing emotional and physical benefits.

Breastfeeding releases hormones such as oxytocin, which can help to promote feelings of relaxation and well-being, as well as reducing stress and anxiety.

For the baby, breastfeeding on demand can help to promote healthy growth and development, as well as providing comfort and security. Breast milk contains all the nutrients a baby needs in the first few months of life, as well as antibodies and other immune-boosting factors that can help to protect against illness and infection. By breastfeeding on demand, the baby is able to get all the benefits of breast milk, ensuring that they are healthy and thriving.

In conclusion, breastfeeding on demand is a beneficial way to prevent plugged ducts and promote good breastfeeding practices.

By allowing the baby to feed whenever they are hungry, the mother can ensure that her breasts are emptied regularly, reducing the risk of blocked ducts and other complications.

Breastfeeding on demand also has a number of other benefits for both mother and baby, including promoting bonding, emotional well-being, and healthy growth and development. Overall, breastfeeding on demand is a natural and effective way to nourish a baby and ensure their health and well-being.

The Importance of Proper Breast Pumping Techniques in Preventing Plugged Ducts

Breastfeeding is a beautiful and natural process that provides numerous benefits for both the mother and the baby. However, for some women, the experience of breastfeeding can be marred by the development of plugged ducts.

Plugged ducts occur when milk flow is obstructed in the breast, leading to pain, swelling, and potential infection. This can be a frustrating and uncomfortable experience for any breastfeeding mother.

One of the key factors that can contribute to the development of plugged ducts is improper breast pumping techniques.

Proper breast pumping techniques are essential for maintaining a healthy milk supply, preventing engorgement, and reducing the risk of plugged ducts.

In this article, we will explore the importance of proper breast pumping techniques in preventing plugged ducts and provide some tips for ensuring a successful breastfeeding experience.

Proper breast pumping techniques are essential for maintaining a healthy milk supply. When a mother pumps her breasts, she is signaling to her body that more milk is needed.

This helps to stimulate milk production and ensure that the baby is adequately nourished. If a mother does not pump her breasts regularly or effectively, she may experience a decrease in milk supply, which can lead to engorgement and potentially plugged ducts.

In addition to maintaining a healthy milk supply, proper breast pumping techniques can also help prevent engorgement.

Engorgement occurs when the breasts become overly full of milk, causing them to feel swollen, tender, and painful. This can make it difficult for the baby to latch on properly and can increase the risk of plugged ducts. By pumping regularly and effectively, a mother can help to prevent engorgement and keep her milk flowing smoothly.

Proper breast pumping techniques can also help to reduce the risk of plugged ducts. Plugged ducts occur when milk flow is obstructed in the breast, leading to pain, swelling, and potential infection.

This can be a painful and uncomfortable experience for any breastfeeding mother.

By using proper breast pumping techniques, a mother can help to ensure that her milk flows freely and that her breasts remain healthy and infection-free.

So, what are some tips for ensuring proper breast pumping techniques? First and foremost, it is important to invest in a high-quality breast pump.

A good breast pump can make all the difference in ensuring a successful breastfeeding experience. Look for a pump that is comfortable, efficient, and easy to use.

There are many different types of breast pumps available on the market, so be sure to do your research and choose one that meets your needs.

Once you have chosen a breast pump, it is important to establish a regular pumping schedule. This will help to maintain a healthy milk supply and prevent engorgement.

Try to pump at least every 2-3 hours during the day and once during the night. It is also important to empty your breasts fully during each pumping session to ensure that your milk flows freely and that your breasts remain healthy.

When pumping, be sure to use the correct flange size for your breasts. The flange is the part of the breast pump that fits over the nipple and areola. Using the correct flange size can help to ensure that your milk flows freely and that your breasts are properly stimulated. If you are unsure of the correct flange size for your breasts, consult with a lactation consultant or breastfeeding specialist.

It is also important to use proper pumping techniques when

expressing milk. Start by massaging your breasts gently to help stimulate milk flow.

Then, position the breast pump over your breast and turn it on. Use a gentle suction setting to avoid discomfort and ensure that your milk flows smoothly. Be sure to pump for at least 15-20 minutes on each breast to ensure that they are fully emptied.

After pumping, be sure to store your breast milk properly. Breast milk can be stored in the refrigerator for up to 4 days or in the freezer for up to 6 months.

Be sure to label your breast milk with the date it was expressed to ensure that it is used in a timely manner. When feeding your baby, be sure to thaw frozen breast milk in the refrigerator or under warm running water.

Do not microwave breast milk, as this can destroy important nutrients and antibodies.

In addition to proper pumping techniques, there are some other steps that you can take to prevent plugged ducts. Be sure to drink plenty of water and eat a healthy, balanced diet to ensure that your body has the nutrients it needs to produce milk.

Avoid tight-fitting bras or clothing that can constrict milk flow. Be sure to get plenty of rest and avoid stress, as these can also affect milk production.

If you do develop a plugged duct, there are some steps that you can take to help clear it. Start by applying a warm compress to the affected breast to help stimulate milk flow. Then, massage the affected area gently to help break up the blockage. You can also try expressing milk by hand or using a breast pump to help clear the duct.

Chapter 9: How to Manage Plugged Milk Ducts While Traveling

Addressing plugged milk ducts while traveling presents a significant challenge for breastfeeding mothers, necessitating prompt attention to prevent complications like mastitis. In this guide, we'll explore effective tips and strategies for managing plugged milk ducts while on the go.

1. Understand the Causes of Plugged Milk Ducts

Plugged milk ducts arise when milk remains inadequately removed from the breast, resulting in duct blockage. Several factors contribute to this, including:

- Infrequent or irregular breastfeeding or pumping.
- Pressure on the breast from tight clothing or an ill-fitting bra.
- Stress, fatigue, or dehydration.
- Poor latch or positioning during breastfeeding.
- Engorgement.

Understanding these causes empowers you to take preventative measures while traveling.

2. Maintain a Consistent Breastfeeding or Pumping Schedule

Consistency in breastfeeding or pumping schedules stands as a key preventive measure against plugged milk ducts while traveling. This practice ensures effective milk removal from the breast, minimizing the risk of blockages.

If traveling across time zones, gradually adjust your breastfeeding or pumping schedule to mitigate sudden changes that could trigger plugged ducts. Additionally, consider increasing the frequency of pumping or breastfeeding to prevent engorgement and ensure optimal milk removal.

3. Stay Hydrated and Maintain a Balanced Diet

Hydration and nutrition play pivotal roles in preventing plugged milk ducts while traveling. Dehydration can lead to denser, more concentrated milk prone to causing duct blockages. Therefore, prioritize ample water intake throughout the day and maintain a diet rich in fruits, vegetables, and whole grains.

To mitigate plugged milk ducts while traveling, it's vital to limit excessive caffeine and alcohol intake, as these substances can dehydrate the body and impact milk production. When traveling to areas with limited access to clean water, consider packing a portable water filter or purchasing bottled water to maintain hydration.

1. Utilize Heat and Massage Techniques for Relief

In the event of a plugged milk duct during travel, several strategies can offer relief. Applying heat to the affected breast can help loosen the blockage and enhance milk flow. Utilize a warm compress like a heated washcloth or heating pad, or opt for a warm shower to alleviate discomfort.

In addition, gentle massage proves beneficial for alleviating plugged milk ducts. Using your fingertips, massage the affected area in circular motions directed towards the nipple. This aids in breaking up the blockage and promoting milk flow. Incorporating massage while breastfeeding or pumping can also aid in duct clearance.

2. Ensure Correct Latch and Positioning

Proper latch and positioning are paramount for effective breastfeeding and serve as preventive measures against plugged milk ducts. Inadequate latch can result in incomplete milk removal, elevating the risk of duct blockages.

Ensure your baby latches deeply onto the breast, covering as much of the areola as possible, to support optimal milk flow and minimize the likelihood of plugged ducts.

When utilizing a breast pump during travel, ensure proper flange size and suction level to avoid discomfort and prevent plugged milk ducts. Ill-fitting flanges or excessive suction can lead to issues. Seek assistance from a lactation consultant or breastfeeding support group if unsure about latch or positioning.

1: Explore Natural Remedies

Several natural remedies can alleviate plugged milk ducts while traveling. Lecithin, a supplement, aids in reducing breast milk viscosity and preventing duct blockages. Consult a healthcare provider before supplementing, especially while breastfeeding. Another remedy is chilled cabbage leaves, which reduce inflammation and discomfort. Simply chill washed and dried cabbage leaves, then apply to the breast for 20-30 minutes.

2. Seek Prompt Medical Attention

If unable to resolve a plugged milk duct independently while traveling or experiencing symptoms like fever, chills, or breast redness and warmth suggestive of mastitis, promptly seek medical attention.

Mastitis requires antibiotics for treatment, and delaying care can lead to complications. When traveling internationally, consider seeking care at local healthcare facilities accustomed to treating breastfeeding mothers.

In conclusion, managing plugged milk ducts during travel poses challenges.

The Benefits of Regular Breast Exams in Preventing Plugged Ducts

Breastfeeding is a beautiful and natural way to nourish your baby, but it can also come with its own set of challenges. One common issue that many breastfeeding mothers face is plugged ducts.

Plugged ducts occur when a milk duct in the breast becomes blocked, leading to pain, swelling, and even infection if left untreated.

Regular breast exams are an important part of preventing plugged ducts and maintaining overall breast health. By checking your breasts regularly, you can catch any potential issues early on and take steps to prevent them from becoming more serious.

In this article, we will explore the benefits of regular breast exams in preventing plugged ducts and how you can incorporate them into your routine.

One of the main benefits of regular breast exams is early detection. By checking your breasts regularly, you can become familiar with how they look and feel, making it easier to notice any changes that may indicate a problem.

This includes checking for lumps, changes in size or shape, and any unusual discharge from the nipples. By catching these changes early, you can seek medical attention promptly and prevent more serious issues from developing.

Regular breast exams can also help you become more aware of your breast health overall. By taking the time to examine your breasts regularly, you can become more in tune with your body and notice any changes that may occur.

This can help you feel more empowered and in control of your health, as you are actively taking steps to monitor and maintain it.

In addition to early detection, regular breast exams can also help prevent plugged ducts specifically. By checking your breasts regularly, you can identify any areas of tenderness or swelling that may indicate a plugged duct forming.

By addressing these issues early on, such as by massaging the affected area or applying warm compresses, you can help prevent the duct from becoming fully blocked and reduce the risk of developing a more serious infection.

Furthermore, regular breast exams can help you establish a baseline for your breast health. By checking your breasts regularly and keeping track of any changes you notice, you can create a record of what is normal for you.

This can be helpful for your healthcare provider if you ever need to seek medical attention for a breast concern, as they can compare any changes to your baseline and determine if further evaluation is needed.

It is important to note that regular breast exams should be part of a comprehensive approach to breast health. In addition to self-exams, it is recommended that women receive regular clinical breast exams by a healthcare provider and mammograms as recommended by their age and risk factors.

These additional screenings can help detect any potential issues that may not be noticeable during a self-exam and provide a more thorough assessment of breast health.

In conclusion, regular breast exams are an important part of preventing plugged ducts and maintaining overall breast health.

By checking your breasts regularly, you can detect any changes early, become more aware of your breast health, prevent plugged ducts, establish a baseline for your breast health, and take control of your well- being.

Incorporating regular breast exams into your routine can help you stay proactive about your health and ensure that you are taking the necessary steps to keep your breasts healthy and functioning optimally.

Remember, early detection is key, so make sure to prioritize regular breast exams as part of your self-care routine.

The Connection Between Breastfeeding Frequency and Plugged Ducts

Breastfeeding is a natural and beneficial way to nourish and bond with your baby. However, it can also come with its challenges, one of which is plugged ducts.

Plugged ducts occur when milk flow is obstructed in the breast, leading to pain, swelling, and a hard lump in the affected area.

This can be a painful and frustrating experience for breastfeeding mothers, but understanding the connection between breastfeeding frequency and plugged ducts can help prevent and manage this common issue.

Breastfeeding frequency refers to how often a mother feeds her baby at the breast. It plays a crucial role in maintaining milk supply and preventing engorgement, which can lead to plugged ducts.

When a mother breastfeeds infrequently, her breasts may become engorged with milk, putting pressure on the milk ducts and increasing the risk of blockages.

On the other hand, breastfeeding too frequently can also lead to plugged ducts, as the breasts may not have enough time to fully empty between feedings.

So, what is the optimal breastfeeding frequency to prevent plugged ducts? The answer may vary from mother to mother, as every woman's body responds differently to breastfeeding.

However, a general guideline is to breastfeed at least 8-12 times a day in the first few weeks after giving birth. This frequent feeding helps establish milk supply and prevents engorgement, reducing the risk of plugged ducts.

As the baby grows and becomes more efficient at breastfeeding, the frequency of feedings may decrease, but it is still important to nurse on demand and empty the breasts fully to prevent blockages.

In addition to breastfeeding frequency, proper positioning and latch are also important factors in preventing plugged ducts. A shallow latch or improper positioning can lead to ineffective milk removal, increasing the risk of blockages.

Mothers should ensure that their baby is latched on correctly and that they are using different breastfeeding positions to fully empty all areas of the breast.

Massaging the breast before and during feedings can also help prevent plugged ducts by promoting milk flow and preventing milk stasis.

If a mother does develop a plugged duct, there are several ways to manage the issue and prevent it from escalating into a more serious condition, such as mastitis.

One of the most effective ways to clear a plugged duct is through frequent nursing or pumping. By emptying the affected breast frequently, the blockage can be loosened and eventually cleared.

Heat therapy, such as warm compresses or a warm shower, can also help alleviate pain and promote milk flow. Massaging the affected area towards the nipple can further aid in clearing the blockage.

In some cases, a mother may need to seek additional treatment for a stubborn plugged duct. Lecithin supplements have been shown to help prevent and manage plugged ducts by reducing the stickiness of breast milk, making it easier for milk to flow freely.

Over-the-counter pain relievers can also help alleviate discomfort associated with plugged ducts. If the blockage does not clear or if the mother develops symptoms of mastitis, such as fever and flu-like symptoms, she should seek medical attention promptly.

It is important for breastfeeding mothers to prioritize their own health and well-being, as plugged ducts can be a painful and disruptive experience.

By understanding the connection between breastfeeding frequency and plugged ducts, mothers can take proactive steps to prevent and manage this common issue.

 Breastfeeding on demand, ensuring proper positioning and latch, and seeking treatment promptly if a plugged duct occurs are all essential strategies for maintaining a healthy breastfeeding relationship with your baby.

Remember, breastfeeding should be a positive and rewarding experience for both mother and baby, and with the right support and knowledge, plugged ducts can be effectively managed.

Chapter 10: The Impact of Medications on Milk Production and Duct Health

Breastfeeding is a natural and invaluable process for both mother and baby, offering crucial nutrients and antibodies for the infant's well-being. However, navigating medication use while breastfeeding can present challenges, particularly concerning milk production and duct health.

The impact of medications on breastfeeding mothers' milk supply and duct health is a significant concern. Certain medications may hinder milk production or compromise the health of milk ducts, potentially leading to complications like mastitis or blocked ducts.

Breastfeeding mothers must stay informed about the potential effects of medications on their lactation and duct health. Collaborating closely with healthcare providers is essential to identify safe and effective solutions tailored to individual needs.

Medications that can disrupt milk production, known as galactagogues, include various types:

- Birth control pills: Some formulations containing hormones can interfere with milk production. Mothers breastfeeding should discuss non-hormonal birth control options with their healthcare providers.

- Decongestants: Certain decongestants, like pseudoephedrine, may diminish milk supply. Breastfeeding mothers experiencing congestion should consult their healthcare providers for alternative solutions that won't compromise lactation.

- Antihistamines: Certain antihistamines may lead to decreased milk production due to their drying effect on the body, including the breasts. Mothers requiring antihistamines should consult their healthcare provider for options compatible with breastfeeding.

- Chemotherapy drugs: Chemotherapy treatments can significantly impact milk production. Mothers undergoing chemotherapy should discuss potential effects on breastfeeding with their healthcare provider and explore alternative feeding options for their infant.

Breastfeeding mothers should communicate any medications they're taking to their healthcare provider to ensure safety for both mother and child.

Medications affecting duct health

Beyond milk production, some medications can influence milk duct health, potentially causing mastitis or blocked ducts, which can be uncomfortable.

Examples include:

- Antidepressants: Certain antidepressants may reduce milk supply and thicken milk, potentially leading to blocked ducts. Mothers taking antidepressants should discuss potential effects on breastfeeding with their healthcare provider and consider alternative treatments if necessary.

- Hormone replacement therapy: This therapy may negatively impact duct health. Mothers using hormone replacement therapy should discuss potential effects on breastfeeding with their healthcare provider and consider alternatives if needed.

- Antibiotics: Some antibiotics might reduce milk supply and disrupt breast bacteria balance, increasing the risk of mastitis. Mothers taking antibiotics should consult their healthcare provider regarding potential effects on breastfeeding and alternative treatments.

Breastfeeding mothers should be mindful of medication effects on duct health and collaborate with their healthcare providers to find suitable solutions.

Tips for maintaining milk production and duct health while on medication

Although certain medications can affect milk production and duct health negatively, breastfeeding mothers can take measures to support milk supply and duct health:

- Stay hydrated: Adequate water intake is vital for maintaining milk production and preventing issues like blocked ducts. Breastfeeding mothers should aim for at least eight glasses of water daily to stay hydrated.

Ensuring proper nutrition, adequate rest, and seeking support are vital for maintaining milk production and duct health while breastfeeding, especially when medications are involved.

1. Nourish with a balanced diet: Consuming a diverse range of nutrient-rich foods, including fruits, vegetables, whole grains, and lean proteins, supports milk production and overall breast health.

2. Prioritize rest: Sufficient rest is crucial for milk production and duct health. Breastfeeding mothers should prioritize adequate rest, both during the day and at night, to promote overall well-being.

3. Seek assistance: Breastfeeding can present challenges, particularly when medications may impact milk production and duct health. Seeking guidance from healthcare providers, lactation consultants, and fellow breastfeeding mothers can offer valuable support in navigating any arising issues.

In summary, understanding how medications may influence milk production and duct health is essential for breastfeeding mothers. While some medications may diminish milk supply or affect duct health negatively, proactive measures such as maintaining a balanced diet, prioritizing rest, and seeking support can help mitigate potential challenges.

The Link Between Allergies and Plugged Milk Ducts

Allergies and plugged milk ducts are two common issues that can affect breastfeeding mothers. While they may seem unrelated, there is actually a link between the two that many women may not be aware of.

In this article, we will explore the connection between allergies and plugged milk ducts, as well as provide tips on how to manage both conditions while breastfeeding.

Allergies are immune system reactions to substances that are normally harmless to most people. Common allergens include pollen, dust mites, pet dander, and certain foods.

Allergies can cause a wide range of symptoms, including sneezing, itching, hives, and in severe cases, anaphylaxis. Allergies can also affect breastfeeding mothers, leading to issues such as plugged milk ducts.

Plugged milk ducts occur when milk is not properly drained from the breast, causing a blockage in the milk duct. This can result in pain, swelling, and redness in the affected breast.

Plugged milk ducts are common among breastfeeding mothers, and can be caused by factors such as poor latching, infrequent feedings, tight clothing, and stress.

So, what is the link between allergies and plugged milk ducts?

Allergies can lead to inflammation in the body, which can in turn affect the milk ducts in the breasts.

When the milk ducts become inflamed, they are more likely to become blocked, leading to plugged milk ducts. Additionally, allergies can also cause changes in the composition of breast milk, which can further contribute to plugged ducts.

If you are a breastfeeding mother with allergies, it is important to be aware of the potential link between allergies and plugged milk ducts. Here are some tips on how to manage both conditions:

1.   Identify and avoid allergens: If you suspect that your allergies are contributing to plugged milk ducts, try to identify and avoid the allergens that trigger your symptoms. This may involve making changes to your diet, avoiding certain foods, or using air purifiers in your home.

2.   Maintain good breastfeeding practices: To prevent plugged milk ducts, it is important to maintain good breastfeeding practices.

This includes ensuring that your baby is latched properly, feeding frequently, and emptying both breasts during each feeding. You can also try different breastfeeding positions to help drain the milk ducts more effectively.

3.   Manage your allergies: If you are experiencing allergy

symptoms, it is important to manage them effectively. This may involve taking antihistamines, using nasal sprays, or avoiding triggers. By managing your allergies, you can help reduce inflammation in your body and lower the risk of plugged milk ducts.

4.	Use heat and massage: If you do develop a plugged milk duct, you can use heat and massage to help clear the blockage. Applying a warm compress to the affected breast and gently massaging the area can help to loosen the blockage and promote milk flow. You can also try using a breast pump or hand expressing to help clear the duct.

5.	Seek support: If you are struggling with allergies and plugged milk ducts, don't hesitate to seek support from a lactation consultant or healthcare provider. They can provide guidance on managing both conditions and offer personalized advice to help you continue breastfeeding successfully.

In conclusion, there is a link between allergies and plugged milk ducts in breastfeeding mothers. By understanding this connection and taking proactive steps to manage both conditions, you can continue to breastfeed your baby successfully.

Remember to identify and avoid allergens, maintain good breastfeeding practices, manage your allergies effectively, use heat and massage to clear plugged ducts, and seek support when needed. With the right approach, you can overcome the challenges of allergies and plugged milk ducts and enjoy a positive breastfeeding experience.

The Role of Blocked Nipples in Plugged Ducts

Blocked nipples and plugged ducts are frequent challenges encountered by breastfeeding mothers, often underestimated in their impact on nursing comfort and effectiveness. Understanding the correlation between blocked nipples and plugged ducts is pivotal for both prevention and treatment of these issues.

Blocked nipples arise when milk ducts become obstructed, impeding the free flow of milk. Various factors contribute to this, such as improper latching, engorgement, or accumulation of dried milk on the nipple.

When a nipple is obstructed, it can culminate in a plugged duct, where milk is trapped within the duct, hindering its natural flow. Consequently, this engenders discomfort, swelling, and inflammation in the breast, thus compromising breastfeeding comfort and potentially escalating to more severe conditions like mastitis.

Central to the interplay between blocked nipples and plugged ducts is the disruption of milk flow. With a blocked nipple, milk encounters obstruction in the duct, resulting in its accumulation and subsequent pressure-induced inflammation, precipitating duct plugging.

Once a duct is occluded, milk passage is impeded, exacerbating discomfort and posing further complications.

Additionally, blocked nipples can exacerbate plugged ducts by impeding milk exit from the breast, causing milk backup in the duct. This accumulation creates a blockage impeding milk flow, intensifying pressure and inflammation, exacerbating the plugged duct.

This vicious cycle can escalate issues, potentially leading to more serious complications.

Understanding this dynamic relationship between blocked nipples and plugged ducts is essential for effective prevention and management, ensuring optimal breastfeeding comfort and health for both mother and baby.

Blocked nipples not only contribute to plugged ducts but can also lead to mastitis, an infection of the breast tissue. Mastitis arises when milk becomes trapped due to blocked nipples, creating an environment conducive to bacterial growth. This infection manifests as pain, swelling, and redness in the affected breast and requires medical attention if left untreated.

Preventing and addressing blocked nipples is paramount for averting plugged ducts and related breastfeeding complications. Ensuring proper latching during breastfeeding is pivotal, facilitating unhindered milk flow through the breast and reducing the likelihood of blockages.

Additionally, maintaining clean, dry nipples mitigates the risk of dried milk buildup that may culminate in blockages.

Treatment for blocked nipples entails various approaches to alleviate discomfort and forestall the onset of plugged ducts.

Applying warm compresses aids in softening the blockage and stimulating milk flow, while gentle breast massage can disperse the obstruction.

Utilizing a breast pump or hand expressing milk can further assist in clearing the blockage and alleviating discomfort.

In instances where blocked nipples persist, more comprehensive interventions may be necessary, such as employing a nipple shield or consulting a lactation consultant.

Nipple shields offer protection and encourage optimal latch, diminishing blockage occurrence. Lactation consultants furnish guidance on correct breastfeeding techniques and address underlying issues contributing to blocked nipples.

In summary, recognizing the association between blocked nipples and plugged ducts is pivotal for effective prevention and treatment. By proactively averting blocked nipples and promptly addressing occurrences, breastfeeding mothers can sidestep discomfort and complications, ensuring successful breastfeeding journeys.

Chapter11: The Benefits of Warm Compresses in Clearing Plugged Milk Ducts

Breastfeeding is a natural and cherished bonding experience between mother and baby, yet it can present challenges like plugged milk ducts. These obstructions in milk flow can cause discomfort, but relief is possible, with warm compresses being a valuable tool.

What exactly are plugged milk ducts?

Plugged milk ducts arise when a milk duct becomes blocked, impeding the flow of milk and resulting in a backlog behind the obstruction. This leads to tenderness, swelling, and inflammation in the affected breast—a common hurdle for breastfeeding mothers, particularly in the initial stages of nursing.

What triggers plugged milk ducts?

Several factors contribute to plugged milk ducts, including:

- Inadequate latch or positioning during breastfeeding
- Constrictive clothing
- Milk oversupply or engorgement
- Pressure on the breast from garments or sleeping positions
- Stress or fatigue

How do warm compresses assist?

Warm compresses offer a straightforward yet effective solution for clearing plugged milk ducts. The warmth aids in softening the blockage, enhancing blood circulation in the area, and facilitating milk flow. This not only eases discomfort but also diminishes inflammation, ultimately resolving the plugged duct.

Advantages of Employing Warm Compresses for Plugged Milk Ducts

Utilizing warm compresses for plugged milk ducts offers numerous benefits, such as:

1. Pain Alleviation: The warmth from warm compresses can effectively ease the discomfort associated with plugged milk ducts.
2. Enhanced Milk Flow: Warm compresses stimulate blood circulation in the affected area, aiding in clearing the blockage and boosting milk flow.

3. Inflammation Reduction: Warm compresses help diminish inflammation in the breast tissue, diminishing pain and swelling.

4. Relaxation: Applying a warm compress provides a soothing experience for nursing mothers, promoting relaxation and stress reduction, which further aids in milk flow.

How to Utilize Warm Compresses for Plugged Milk Ducts

Employing warm compresses for plugged milk ducts is straightforward. Follow these steps:

1. Begin by saturating a clean washcloth in warm water, ensuring it's not too hot to prevent skin burns.

2. Gently wring out excess water from the washcloth and place it on the affected breast.

3. Leave the warm compress on the breast for 10-15 minutes or until it cools down.

4. Repeat this process multiple times daily until the plugged duct clears.

Tips for Maximizing Warm Compress Effectiveness

- Utilize a warm shower or bath as an alternative method to clear plugged milk ducts by allowing warm water to run over the breasts for a few minutes.

- Consider using a warm rice sock or microwavable heating pad for convenience and effective heat application.

- Massage the affected breast while using the warm compress to further promote milk flow and blockage clearance.

- If pain persists or the plugged duct doesn't clear within a few days, seek advice from a healthcare provider promptly.

In summary, integrating warm compresses into your breastfeeding routine can significantly aid in managing plugged milk ducts. By leveraging the benefits of heat to enhance blood flow, diminish inflammation, and increase milk flow, warm compresses offer relief from discomfort and support a comfortable nursing experience.

The Connection Between Clogged Milk Ducts and Breast Infections

Breastfeeding embodies natural beauty and confers numerous advantages for both mother and child. Yet, like many aspects of motherhood, it presents its own hurdles. Among these challenges, clogged milk ducts stand out as a common issue, potentially escalating into more severe complications such as breast infections.

Clogged milk ducts occur when milk flow within the breast becomes obstructed, resulting in a buildup of milk. Various factors contribute to this blockage, including improper latching, irregular breastfeeding or pumping, constraining attire, and even stress.

When a milk duct becomes obstructed, it triggers pain, swelling, and redness in the affected breast. Left unaddressed, clogged ducts can progress into mastitis, a condition characterized by inflammation of breast tissue, often instigated by bacterial entry through a cracked nipple or obstructed duct.

Symptoms of mastitis encompass fever, chills, body aches, flu-like sensations, alongside the discomfort typical of clogged milk ducts. Prompt medical intervention, including antibiotics, is essential to manage mastitis effectively.

The correlation between clogged milk ducts and breast infections is evident: a blocked duct can foster bacterial growth, culminating in an infection.

Breastfeeding mothers must promptly attend to clogged milk ducts to forestall the development of mastitis. Here are some strategies for preventing and addressing clogged milk ducts:

1. Ensure Proper Latching: Proper latching is paramount for efficient breastfeeding. Inadequate latch increases the likelihood of milk duct blockage. Seek assistance from a lactation consultant if encountering difficulties with latching.

1. Breastfeed Frequently: Maintaining a regular breastfeeding schedule is essential for promoting smooth milk flow and preventing milk duct blockages. Strive to breastfeed every 2-3 hours during the day and include at least one feeding session at night.

2. Explore Different Breastfeeding Positions: Experimenting with various breastfeeding positions can aid in effectively draining all areas of the breast.

Discovering positions that suit both you and your baby can optimize milk flow.

3. Gentle Breast Massage: Incorporating gentle massage techniques on the affected breast can help alleviate blockages and stimulate milk flow. This can be done during breastfeeding, pumping sessions, or while enjoying a warm shower.

4. Apply Heat: Using warm compresses on the affected breast can alleviate discomfort and encourage milk flow. Whether it's a warm washcloth or a heating pad, applying heat can provide relief.

5. Maintain Hydration and Nutrition: Adequate hydration and a balanced diet are crucial for sustaining milk production and preventing clogged milk ducts.

If you encounter a clogged milk duct, here are steps to aid in its clearance:

1. Continue Breastfeeding: Continuing to breastfeed is paramount for resolving a clogged duct. Ensure frequent nursing on the affected breast and verify proper latching to facilitate milk flow.

1. Apply Cold Therapy: Using cold packs can effectively reduce swelling and alleviate discomfort. Apply a cold pack to the affected area for 15-20 minutes multiple times a day to experience relief.

2. Utilize Over-the-Counter Pain Relievers: Over-the-counter pain relievers like ibuprofen or acetaminophen can provide relief from pain and discomfort associated with clogged milk ducts. Ensure you adhere to the recommended dosage guidelines.

3. Prioritize Rest and Relaxation: Stress can exacerbate clogged milk ducts, so it's essential to prioritize relaxation and rest. Allocate time for relaxation techniques, aim for sufficient rest, and consider delegating household tasks and childcare responsibilities.

If persistent symptoms of a clogged milk duct persist beyond 24-48 hours or if signs of mastitis develop, seek prompt medical attention. Consulting your healthcare provider for a proper diagnosis is crucial, as they can recommend suitable treatment options, including antibiotics if necessary.

In summary, clogged milk ducts and subsequent breast infections are common challenges encountered by breastfeeding mothers. By adopting preventive measures and promptly addressing any issues that arise, the risk of developing severe complications such as mastitis can be minimized.

Remember to prioritize self-care, seek assistance when needed, and have confidence in your body's ability to nourish your baby. With adequate support, breastfeeding remains a beautiful and fulfilling journey despite potential obstacles.

The Impact of Inadequate Milk Supply on Plugged Ducts

Breastfeeding is a natural and important part of motherhood. It provides numerous benefits to both the mother and the baby, including bonding, nutrition, and immune system support. However, breastfeeding can sometimes come with its own set of challenges, one of which is inadequate milk supply.

Inadequate milk supply occurs when a mother's breast does not produce enough milk to meet the needs of her baby. This can be caused by a variety of factors, including hormonal imbalances, improper latch, or insufficient milk removal.

When a mother does not have enough milk to feed her baby, it can lead to a range of issues, one of which is plugged ducts.

Plugged ducts are a common problem that can occur when milk is not effectively removed from the breast. This can happen when a baby does not latch properly, or when a mother is not emptying her breasts completely during feedings.

 When milk becomes trapped in the ducts, it can lead to inflammation and blockages, causing pain, swelling, and even infection.

The impact of inadequate milk supply on plugged ducts can be significant. When a mother is not producing enough milk, her baby may not be getting the nutrition they need, leading to poor growth and development.

Additionally, the discomfort and pain caused by plugged ducts can make breastfeeding even more challenging, leading to frustration and stress for both the mother and the baby.

Inadequate milk supply can also have long-term effects on a mother's milk production. When milk is not effectively removed from the breast, it can signal to the body that less milk is needed, leading to a decrease in milk supply over time. This can create a vicious cycle, where plugged ducts lead to decreased milk production, which in turn leads to more plugged ducts.

To prevent the impact of inadequate milk supply on plugged ducts, it is important for mothers to take steps to increase their milk production and ensure effective milk removal.

This can include techniques such as frequent nursing, proper latch, and breast massage to help prevent blockages and keep milk flowing smoothly.

Mothers who are experiencing plugged ducts should also seek support from a lactation consultant or healthcare provider. They can provide guidance on how to effectively remove milk from the breast, as well as offer tips on managing pain and inflammation. In some cases, medication may be necessary to help clear the blockages and prevent infection.

In conclusion, the impact of inadequate milk supply on plugged ducts can be significant and challenging for both mother and baby.

By taking steps to increase milk production and ensure effective milk removal, mothers can help prevent plugged ducts and maintain a healthy breastfeeding relationship with their baby.

Seeking support from a lactation consultant or healthcare provider can also be beneficial in managing plugged ducts and preventing further complications.

Breastfeeding is a beautiful and natural process, and with the right support and guidance, mothers can overcome the challenges of inadequate milk supply and enjoy a positive breastfeeding experience.

Chapter 12: The Benefits of Proper Hydration in Preventing Plugged Ducts

Adequate hydration is not just essential for overall health; it plays a pivotal role in preventing blockages in various ducts throughout the body, whether in the breast, ear, or tear ducts.

These blockages can lead to discomfort, pain, and potentially severe infections if left unaddressed. Prioritizing hydration can significantly mitigate the risk of such blockages and promote optimal bodily function.

One of the primary advantages of staying properly hydrated is its ability to maintain tissue lubrication. Dehydration can render tissues dry and adhesive, facilitating the formation of blockages within ducts. By consuming sufficient water daily, you ensure adequate tissue hydration, thereby reducing the likelihood of blockages.

Moreover, proper hydration facilitates the smooth flow of bodily fluids. When adequately hydrated, fluids move more freely through the ducts, minimizing the probability of blockage formation.

This is particularly crucial for breast ducts, where blockages can escalate into mastitis, a painful breast tissue infection. Consistent hydration promotes fluid movement, preventing blockages and associated complications.

In addition to promoting fluid flow, adequate hydration aids in detoxification. Dehydration heightens the accumulation of toxins and waste products in tissues and ducts, elevating the risk of blockages. By consuming ample water daily, you support the elimination of these toxins, diminishing the likelihood of blockages and maintaining overall bodily health.

Furthermore, hydration is vital for bolstering the immune system. Dehydration compromises immune function, making the body more susceptible to infections.

Since blockages in ducts can harbor bacteria and pathogens, hydration becomes critical in fortifying the immune response and reducing infection risk. Consistent hydration supports immune strength, minimizing the chance of infections stemming from blockages.

In essence, prioritizing hydration not only fosters overall health but also serves as a fundamental strategy in preventing blockages in various body ducts. By ensuring proper hydration, you uphold tissue lubrication, facilitate fluid movement, support detoxification, and bolster immune function, collectively reducing the risk of blockages and associated complications.

Moreover, maintaining proper hydration is paramount for overall health and vitality. Adequate hydration optimizes bodily functions, serving as a crucial preventive measure against various health issues, including plugged ducts.

It fosters improved digestion, regulates body temperature, and facilitates the body's natural detoxification processes. Consistently meeting your body's water needs promotes optimal function, mitigating the risk of plugged ducts and other health concerns.

In summary, ensuring proper hydration is fundamental in preventing plugged ducts within the body. By preserving tissue lubrication, promoting fluid flow, and fortifying the immune system, you can effectively minimize the likelihood of blockages and plugged ducts.

Moreover, maintaining hydration aids in toxin elimination, upholds overall health and wellness, and guards against a spectrum of health issues. Prioritizing hydration in your daily regimen empowers you to sustain bodily health and functionality, reducing the risk of plugged ducts and associated health complications.

The Role of Breastfeeding Support Groups in Preventing Plugged Ducts

Breastfeeding is a natural and beautiful way for mothers to nourish their babies. It provides numerous benefits for both mother and baby, including bonding, immunity, and nutrition. However, breastfeeding can also come with its challenges, one of which is plugged ducts.

Plugged ducts occur when a milk duct in the breast becomes blocked, causing milk to back up and create a painful lump.

This can happen for a variety of reasons, including poor latch, infrequent feeding, tight clothing, or stress. Plugged ducts can be uncomfortable and even painful for breastfeeding mothers, making it important to address them promptly.

Breastfeeding support groups play a crucial role in preventing plugged ducts by providing education, support, and resources for breastfeeding mothers.

These groups bring together women who are going through similar experiences, allowing them to share advice, tips, and encouragement.

By fostering a sense of community and camaraderie, breastfeeding support groups can help mothers navigate the challenges of breastfeeding and avoid common issues like plugged ducts.

One of the key benefits of breastfeeding support groups is the access to knowledgeable and experienced lactation consultants.

These professionals can offer guidance on proper breastfeeding techniques, positioning, and latch to help prevent plugged ducts. They can also provide information on how to recognize the signs of a plugged duct and how to effectively address it.

In addition to lactation consultants, breastfeeding support groups often have peer counselors who have personal experience with breastfeeding.

These women can offer valuable insights and tips based on their own experiences, helping new mothers feel more confident and supported in their breastfeeding journey.

Peer counselors can also provide emotional support and encouragement, which can be invaluable in preventing plugged ducts.

Breastfeeding support groups also provide a platform for mothers to ask questions and seek advice from their peers. By sharing their concerns and challenges, mothers can receive feedback and suggestions from other women who have been in similar situations.

This can help mothers troubleshoot potential issues before they escalate into plugged ducts.

Furthermore, breastfeeding support groups offer a safe and nonjudgmental space for mothers to discuss their breastfeeding experiences. This can be particularly important for women who may be struggling with breastfeeding or feeling overwhelmed.

By providing a supportive environment, breastfeeding support groups can help mothers feel more comfortable seeking help and advice, reducing the likelihood of plugged ducts.

Another important role of breastfeeding support groups in preventing plugged ducts is the promotion of self-care practices.

Breastfeeding can be physically demanding and emotionally draining, making it essential for mothers to prioritize their own well-being.

Support groups can educate mothers on the importance of self-care, including adequate rest, hydration, nutrition, and stress management. By encouraging mothers to take care of themselves, support groups can help prevent plugged ducts and other breastfeeding complications.

Breastfeeding support groups also play a role in advocating for breastfeeding-friendly policies and practices in the community.

By raising awareness about the benefits of breastfeeding and the challenges that mothers may face, support groups can help create a more supportive environment for breastfeeding mothers.

This can include advocating for workplace accommodations, public breastfeeding rights, and access to lactation support services.

 By advocating for breastfeeding-friendly policies, support groups can help reduce the barriers that may contribute to plugged ducts and other breastfeeding issues.

In conclusion, breastfeeding support groups play a vital role in preventing plugged ducts by providing education, support, and resources for breastfeeding mothers.

By offering access to lactation consultants, peer counselors, and a supportive community, these groups can help mothers navigate the challenges of breastfeeding and avoid common issues like plugged ducts.

Through advocacy, education, and self-care promotion, breastfeeding support groups can empower mothers to breastfeed successfully and comfortably. By promoting a positive and supportive breastfeeding environment, support groups can help prevent plugged ducts and other breastfeeding complications, ensuring that mothers and babies can enjoy the many benefits of breastfeeding.

The Connection Between Breast Engorgement and Plugged Ducts

Breast engorgement and plugged ducts are common challenges encountered by breastfeeding mothers. Although distinct, these issues often intertwine, contributing to discomfort and potential complications.

Here, we delve into the causes of both conditions, their correlation, and strategies for prevention and treatment.

Breast engorgement arises when the breasts become excessively full of milk, triggered by various factors like postpartum milk influx, infrequent breastfeeding, or an imbalance between milk production and removal. It manifests as discomfort and swelling and may escalate to complications such as mastitis or plugged ducts if overlooked.

Plugged ducts occur when a milk duct becomes obstructed, hindering milk flow. This obstruction typically arises from inadequate milk removal, stemming from improper latch or infrequent breastfeeding. Plugged ducts entail pain, swelling, and redness, potentially escalating to severe issues if untreated.

The nexus between breast engorgement and plugged ducts lies in the former's propensity to predispose duct blockage.

When breasts are engorged, milk flow through ducts is impeded, heightening the risk of obstruction. Additionally, engorgement induces breast tissue inflammation, exacerbating milk passage difficulties.

Preventing both breast engorgement and plugged ducts involves several measures. Ensuring frequent and effective breastfeeding is paramount. This ensures regular milk removal, mitigating engorgement and blockage risks.

Proper breastfeeding techniques, including optimal latch and varied positions, aid in comprehensive milk extraction, reducing the likelihood of engorgement and plugged ducts.

In essence, breast engorgement and plugged ducts often coalesce, compounding breastfeeding challenges. Understanding their interplay is crucial for effective management. By prioritizing frequent and proper breastfeeding techniques, mothers can diminish the incidence of engorgement and plugged ducts, fostering a smoother breastfeeding journey for both mother and child.

Aside from frequent breastfeeding, mothers have various techniques to prevent engorgement and plugged ducts. Before nursing, applying warm compresses to the breasts can stimulate milk flow, while cold compresses afterward can alleviate swelling and inflammation. Additionally, massaging the breasts during breastfeeding aids in efficient milk removal.

Should engorgement or plugged ducts arise, several measures can ease symptoms and prevent complications. Continuing regular breastfeeding is crucial, ensuring milk removal and potentially clearing blockages. Warm compresses and gentle massage can further promote milk flow and reduce swelling.

If symptoms persist or worsen, seeking medical attention is vital. Healthcare providers can identify underlying causes and recommend appropriate treatments, such as over-the-counter pain relievers, breast pumping, or antibiotics for infections.

In summary, breast engorgement and plugged ducts are common issues for breastfeeding mothers, often interconnected. Through preventive measures like frequent and effective breastfeeding, warm compresses, and prompt medical attention, mothers can reduce their risk of experiencing these discomforting conditions.

Chapter13: The Impact of Illness on Milk Production and Duct Health

Breastfeeding stands as a cornerstone of infant health and development, with the quality and quantity of breast milk directly influencing a baby's growth and well-being. However, various factors, including illness, can impede a mother's ability to produce an ample milk supply.

Illness profoundly affects milk production and duct health in lactating mothers. When a mother falls ill, her body may prioritize allocating resources toward combating the infection or illness rather than sustaining milk production.

Consequently, this redirection can lead to a decrease in milk supply, posing concerns for both the mother and the baby.

Moreover, illness doesn't solely impact milk production; it also affects the health of the milk ducts. Infections, inflammation, and other complications in the ducts may induce pain, discomfort, and potential blockages, further inhibiting milk production.

Recognizing the repercussions of illness on milk production and duct health is crucial for healthcare providers and lactating mothers alike.

The Impact of Illness on Milk Production

Illness directly influences milk production in lactating mothers. When a mother falls ill, her body may prioritize fighting off the infection or illness over producing milk, resulting in a decreased milk supply—a concern shared by both mother and baby.

Furthermore, illness can alter the composition of breast milk. Certain illnesses can modify the levels of nutrients, antibodies, and other beneficial components, thereby affecting the baby's health and development. For instance, a mother with a cold or flu might produce milk enriched with higher antibody levels to safeguard her baby from the illness.

In some instances, illness might halt milk production temporarily. This scenario is particularly worrisome for mothers exclusively breastfeeding their babies. In such cases, it's imperative for healthcare providers to collaborate with the mother to address the underlying illness and provide support to sustain or restore her milk supply.

Impact of Illness on Duct Health

Apart from its effect on milk production, illness can significantly influence the health of milk ducts, vital channels for milk transport from mammary glands to the nipple during breastfeeding. Inflammation, infection, or blockage of these ducts can lead to discomfort and complications for both mother and baby.

Infections within the milk ducts, such as mastitis, present considerable challenges. Mastitis, characterized by bacterial invasion into breast tissue through cracks in the nipple, manifests with swelling, redness, tenderness, and flu-like symptoms like fever and chills.

Mastitis profoundly impacts milk production, as inflammation and infection in the ducts can decrease milk supply and alter milk composition. In severe cases, abscesses may form in breast tissue, necessitating surgical drainage.

Besides mastitis, issues like blocked ducts can also affect milk production and duct health. Blocked ducts occur when milk becomes trapped, causing pain, swelling, and potential infection. If left unaddressed, blocked ducts can escalate to mastitis or other complications, further hindering milk production.

Managing Illness and Its Impact on Milk Production and Duct Health

When a lactating mother falls ill, seeking medical attention is crucial to address the underlying illness. Healthcare providers must consider the medication's effects on milk production and duct health when prescribing treatment.

Alongside medical intervention, several strategies help manage illness and its impact on milk production and duct health. Rest and hydration support the body's immune response and healing. Continuing regular breastfeeding or pumping, even when unwell, helps maintain or restore milk supply.

Warm compresses applied to affected breasts alleviate pain and inflammation in milk ducts. Massage and gentle pressure can clear blocked ducts and encourage milk flow. Lactating mothers should avoid tight clothing or bras that may exacerbate duct issues.

Severe pain, swelling, or concerning symptoms warrant immediate medical attention. Timely treatment of milk duct infections and other issues prevents complications and supports milk production. Healthcare providers may recommend antibiotics, pain relief, or other interventions to address underlying problems.

The Benefits of Massage Oils in Clearing Plugged Milk Ducts

Breastfeeding is a natural and wonderful experience that offers numerous benefits for both mother and baby. However, it comes with its share of challenges, and one common hurdle is dealing with plugged milk ducts.

These obstructions can cause discomfort and, if left unattended, may escalate into more severe issues like mastitis. Fortunately, there are effective methods for clearing plugged milk ducts, with massage oils being a noteworthy option.

Massage oils have a long history of use for their therapeutic qualities and can be particularly helpful in addressing plugged milk ducts. Various types of massage oils are available, each offering unique advantages. Among the popular choices for clearing plugged milk ducts are olive oil, coconut oil, and sweet almond oil.

One primary benefit of using massage oils for this purpose is their ability to diminish inflammation and enhance circulation in the affected area.

Plugged ducts often result in swelling and inflammation, impeding milk flow. By massaging the area with a soothing oil, inflammation can be reduced, and blood flow improved, aiding in clearing the blockage and alleviating discomfort.

Moreover, massage oils contribute to softening the skin, easing milk passage. Plugged ducts can lead to dry, irritated skin surrounding the area, further impeding milk flow. Massage oils nourish the skin, making it more supple, and facilitating milk movement, ultimately aiding in clearing the blockage.

Another advantage of using massage oils is their ability to relax muscles and diminish tension. Plugged milk ducts can cause surrounding muscles to tighten, exacerbating discomfort during breastfeeding.

By massaging the area with a calming oil, muscle tension can be reduced, leading to pain relief and a more pleasant breastfeeding experience.

In addition to the physical benefits, incorporating massage oils into the routine for clearing plugged milk ducts can offer emotional advantages for breastfeeding mothers. Breastfeeding itself can be a demanding and stressful journey, and dealing with plugged ducts can exacerbate these feelings. Taking a moment to massage the affected area with a soothing oil can promote relaxation and tranquility, easing stress and enhancing overall well-being.

When selecting a massage oil for addressing plugged milk ducts, certain considerations should be taken into account. Firstly, prioritize safety by opting for high-quality oils that are organic, cold-pressed, and devoid of additives or preservatives, ensuring they are safe for both you and your baby.

 Popular choices like olive oil, coconut oil, and sweet almond oil are renowned for their gentle and nourishing properties, ideal for the delicate skin of breastfeeding mothers.

Moreover, pay attention to the scent of the oil, as some fragrances may be overwhelming. If you are sensitive to scents, opt for a fragrance-free oil or one with a subtle, natural aroma.

Additionally, consider the texture of the oil and how it feels on your skin. Some oils may leave a greasy residue, while others absorb quickly, providing a luxurious and comfortable sensation during massage.

When employing massage oils to clear plugged milk ducts, adopt gentle, circular motions with light pressure. Begin by massaging the affected area in circular movements, progressing from the breast's periphery towards the nipple.

 Applying gentle pressure aids in dislodging blockages and stimulating milk flow. To enhance effectiveness, precede massage with a warm compress or shower to soften the skin and facilitate blockage clearance.

In addition to massage oils, several other methods can effectively clear plugged milk ducts and prevent their recurrence:

- Nursing frequently: Regular and on-demand breastfeeding empties the breasts, preventing milk stagnation and blockage formation.
- Using a breast pump: For those unable to nurse directly, regular pumping maintains milk flow, preventing blockages.
- Applying heat: Warm compresses or showers soften the skin, easing blockage clearance, reducing inflammation, and enhancing circulation in the affected area.

The Role of Herbal Remedies in Preventing Plugged Ducts

Plugged ducts pose a common challenge for breastfeeding mothers, occurring when milk ducts become obstructed, impeding the smooth flow of milk. This obstruction can result in discomfort, swelling, and inflammation in the affected breast.

While dealing with plugged ducts can be distressing, there are various preventive measures available, with herbal remedies emerging as a promising approach.

Herbal remedies, deeply rooted in traditional medicine, have long been utilized to address a spectrum of health concerns, including breastfeeding-related issues.

Many herbs boast anti-inflammatory, antibacterial, and analgesic properties, rendering them effective in averting and managing plugged ducts. This article seeks to elucidate the role of herbal remedies in thwarting plugged ducts and outline their safe and efficient utilization by breastfeeding mothers.

Understanding the Common Causes of Plugged Ducts

Before delving into the realm of herbal remedies for plugged ducts, it's essential to grasp the prevalent triggers of this condition:

- Inadequate breast emptying: When milk remains incompletely drained during feedings, it fosters milk accumulation within the ducts, heightening the risk of obstruction.

- External pressure on the breasts: Tight undergarments, sleeping positions that compress the breasts, or carrying heavy loads on a single shoulder can exert pressure on the breasts, contributing to duct blockage.

- Suboptimal latch: An improper latch impedes the infant's ability to effectively draw milk from the breast, elevating the likelihood of plugged ducts.

- Stress-induced disruptions: Stress can adversely affect milk production and flow dynamics, predisposing ducts to obstruction.

- Hormonal fluctuations: Changes in hormonal levels, such as those occurring during menstruation or weaning, can disrupt milk production patterns, augmenting the susceptibility to plugged ducts.

Preventing Plugged Ducts Naturally with Herbal Remedies

Harnessing the power of herbal remedies can be an effective strategy in thwarting plugged ducts by nurturing healthy milk flow, curbing inflammation, and bolstering breast health. Below are some potent herbs renowned for their efficacy in preventing plugged ducts:

1. Fenugreek: Widely esteemed for its ability to enhance milk supply and deter plugged ducts, fenugreek boasts anti-inflammatory properties that mitigate breast swelling and optimize milk flow. It can be consumed in capsule form or steeped into a soothing tea.

2. Marshmallow Root: Revered for its calming and anti-inflammatory attributes, marshmallow root aids in quelling breast inflammation and fostering unobstructed milk flow, making it a valuable ally in preventing plugged ducts. It can be brewed into a comforting tea or ingested as capsules.

3. Dandelion Root: Potent in supporting liver function and promoting digestive wellness, dandelion root plays a pivotal role in averting plugged ducts. By ameliorating breast inflammation and optimizing milk flow, it contributes to breast health. Enjoy it as a tea infusion or through capsules.

4. Red Clover: Celebrated for its prowess in fortifying breast health and staving off plugged ducts, red clover's anti-inflammatory properties assuage breast swelling and enhance milk flow. It can be consumed as a fragrant tea or in capsule form.

5. Blessed Thistle: Embraced for its traditional use in augmenting milk supply and thwarting plugged ducts, blessed thistle aids in optimizing milk flow and diminishing breast inflammation. It can be ingested in capsule form or brewed into a comforting tea.

6. Nettle: Rich in vital nutrients, nettle bolsters overall breast health and shields against plugged ducts. Its abundance in vitamins and minerals facilitates optimal milk production and flow. Enjoy it as a fortifying tea or through capsules.

7. Ginger: Revered for its warming properties, ginger enhances circulation and diminishes breast inflammation, thereby deterring plugged ducts. Its soothing effects alleviate discomfort associated with plugged ducts. Enjoy it as a comforting tea or incorporate it into culinary delights.

8. Echinacea: Potent in fortifying the immune system and quelling breast inflammation, echinacea stands as a stalwart guardian against plugged ducts. It combats infections that may precipitate duct blockages. It can be

consumed in capsule form or brewed into a revitalizing tea.

Ensuring the Safe Utilization of Herbal Remedies to Prevent Plugged Ducts

Employing herbal remedies for averting plugged ducts can indeed be beneficial, yet their usage should be approached with caution and prudence. Here are some guidelines to ensure their safe and responsible utilization:

- Seek guidance from a healthcare professional: Prior to integrating any herbal remedies into your regimen, seek counsel from a healthcare professional, particularly if you are pregnant, lactating, or have existing health concerns.

- Opt for premium-grade herbs: When procuring herbal remedies, prioritize those sourced from reputable suppliers and certified organic sources. This ensures their purity, potency, and safety for consumption.

Chapter14: The Connection Between Plugged Milk Ducts and Breastfeeding Success

Breastfeeding embodies a natural and enriching journey for both mother and baby, yet it often presents challenges. One such challenge is the occurrence of plugged milk ducts, disrupting this otherwise seamless process.

Despite their discomfort, with appropriate insights and methods, plugged milk ducts can be effectively addressed, ensuring continued success in breastfeeding.

Within this comprehensive guide, we delve into the correlation between plugged milk ducts and breastfeeding triumphs. Furthermore, we furnish a detailed roadmap for unblocking impediments, thus guaranteeing a harmonious breastfeeding voyage for mother and baby alike.

Understanding Plugged Milk Ducts

Plugged milk ducts ensue when milk flow encounters hindrances within the duct, resulting in milk accumulation behind the barrier. This manifests as pain, swelling, and inflammation in the affected breast. A prevalent issue among breastfeeding mothers, plugged milk ducts stem from various factors, including:

- Improper latch or positioning during breastfeeding
- Inadequate breast emptying, either infrequently or incompletely
- External pressure on the breast from ill-fitting attire or undergarments
- Stress or exhaustion
- Mastitis, an infection affecting the breast tissue

Symptoms of plugged milk ducts typically include.
- Highlighting the Symptoms of Plugged Milk Ducts

Plugged milk ducts typically manifest through various symptoms, including:

- The presence of a small, tender lump within the breast
- Pain or discomfort experienced in the affected breast
- Swelling or redness observed in the affected area
- A sensation of fullness or heaviness felt in the breast
- A reduction in milk supply from the affected breast

Addressing Plugged Milk Ducts for Continued Breastfeeding Success

Timely intervention is crucial in addressing plugged milk ducts to mitigate further complications, such as mastitis or a decline in milk production. By recognizing the correlation between plugged milk ducts and breastfeeding triumphs, mothers can proactively undertake measures to alleviate the blockage, thus facilitating successful breastfeeding.

Understanding the Impact of Plugged Milk Ducts on Breastfeeding Success

Plugged milk ducts pose a significant hurdle to breastfeeding success. These obstructions disrupt milk flow, resulting in discomfort and diminished milk output in the affected breast.

Consequently, breastfeeding becomes a painful and challenging experience for both mother and baby, potentially leading to premature weaning if left unattended.

Beyond the physical discomfort, plugged milk ducts also take a toll on a mother's mental and emotional well-being. Breastfeeding embodies a deeply personal and emotionally charged journey for many women. Thus, encountering obstacles like plugged milk ducts can evoke feelings of discouragement and despair.

 It is imperative for breastfeeding mothers to seek assistance and guidance in navigating such challenges to ensure a positive and rewarding breastfeeding journey.

Clearing Plugged Milk Ducts: A Comprehensive Guide

Dealing with plugged milk ducts can be challenging, but there are effective techniques to restore milk flow and continue breastfeeding successfully. Follow these steps to clear the path and ensure a smooth breastfeeding journey:

1. Breastfeed frequently and effectively: Ensure proper latching and nurse on demand to empty the affected breast thoroughly. Start nursing sessions with the affected breast to encourage milk flow and prevent further blockages.

2. Apply heat: Ease discomfort and encourage milk flow by applying a warm compress for 10-15 minutes before nursing or pumping. Heat helps soften the blockage, making it easier to clear.

3. Massage the affected breast: Use gentle circular motions and pressure to massage the blocked area, moving towards the nipple. Massage before nursing or pumping to break up the blockage and aid in emptying the breast.

4. Try different nursing positions: Experiment with various positions like the football hold, cradle hold, or side-lying position to ensure complete breast emptying and promote milk flow.

5. Utilize a breast pump: If nursing alone isn't sufficient, use a breast pump after nursing sessions to fully empty the breast. Opt for a gentle suction setting to avoid further irritation and effectively clear plugged ducts.

6. Maintain hydration and nutrition: Stay adequately hydrated and nourished to support your body during this process. Proper hydration and nutrition are essential for overall breast health and milk production.

By following these steps, breastfeeding mothers can effectively address plugged milk ducts and maintain a successful breastfeeding journey.

Conclusion

In closing, **"Mastering Plugged Ducts in Breastfeeding: A Complete Manual for Prevention and Remedy"** empowers you with expert insights, practical strategies, and nurturing remedies to reclaim the joy of breastfeeding without the hindrance of blocked ducts.

Throughout this journey, we've delved into the causes of plugged ducts, explored effective prevention methods, and discovered powerful techniques for clearing them.

From frequent nursing to applying heat, from utilizing herbal remedies to seeking professional guidance, you now possess a wealth of knowledge to navigate through any challenges that may arise in your breastfeeding journey.

As you unleash the power of your maternal journey, remember that you are not alone. With the tools provided in this guide, you can overcome obstacles with confidence and grace. Let "Unblocking the Path" be your ultimate companion on the road to seamless lactation, ensuring that every moment spent nourishing your little one is filled with comfort, joy, and fulfillment.

Embrace this journey with determination, knowing that you have the resources and support to overcome any hurdles that may come your way. Your dedication to providing the best for your baby is unwavering, and with the guidance offered in this book, you are equipped to flourish in your role as a breastfeeding mother.

Discover the power within you, embrace the journey ahead, and let "Unblocking the Path" be your guiding light towards a fulfilling and rewarding breastfeeding experience. Together, let us celebrate the beauty of motherhood and the boundless love we share with our precious little ones.

Biography

Introducing **Alice Brendan**, a passionate advocate for maternal wellness and the author behind the empowering book **"Mastering Plugged Ducts in Breastfeeding: A Complete Manual for Prevention and Remedy."**

With a background in maternal health and lactation consulting, Alice brings a wealth of expertise and firsthand experience to her writing. Her journey into the world of breastfeeding began as a mother herself, navigating the challenges and triumphs of breastfeeding her own children.

Inspired by her personal journey and driven by a desire to support other mothers on their path to breastfeeding success, Alice embarked on a mission to empower women with the knowledge and tools they need to overcome common breastfeeding obstacles.

Drawing on her extensive research and practical experience, Alice provides insightful guidance and actionable strategies for preventing and treating plugged milk ducts, ensuring a seamless and joyful breastfeeding experience for mothers and babies alike.

Her compassionate approach and unwavering dedication to maternal wellness shine through in every page of her ebook, offering a beacon of hope and encouragement to mothers facing breastfeeding challenges.

When she's not writing or supporting mothers on their breastfeeding journey, Alice can be found indulging in her love for nature walks, yoga, and spending quality time with her family.

Her nurturing spirit and genuine passion for empowering mothers radiate through her work, making her an invaluable resource for mothers seeking support and guidance on their breastfeeding journey.

Join Alice on a transformative journey of empowerment and discovery as you embark on the path to breastfeeding bliss. With "Liberate Your Lactation" as your guide, you'll unlock the secrets to overcoming plugged milk ducts and embracing the transformative power of breastfeeding with confidence and ease.